D0409748

TINNITUS

By the same author

TINNITUS – LEARNING TO LIVE WITH IT

Published by Ashgrove Press, Bath
First Published in Great Britain 1987
Second Printing 1989
USA Distribution Avery Publishing, New York

ISBN 0-906798-80-9

TINNITUS

by

LESLIE SHEPPARD

edited by

DR CLIVE SHEPPARD
MA, MB, BChir(Camb), MRCGP

PUBLISHED THROUGH THE NORFOLK
TINNITUS SOCIETY
Wingfield Lower Gresham
Norfolk NR11 8RE
Tel: 026 377 285

Registered Charity No 1005309

First Published 1993 in Great Britain
through
The Norfolk Tinnitus Society
Wingfield, Lower Gresham
Norfolk NR11 8RE

British Library Cataloguing-in-Publication Data
A catalogue record for this book is available
from the British Library

ISBN 0-9520642-1-9

Cover Logo by Joanne Radmilovich by permission of
The American Tinnitus Association

Typeset, printed and bound in Great Britain by
Page Bros, Norwich

CONTENTS

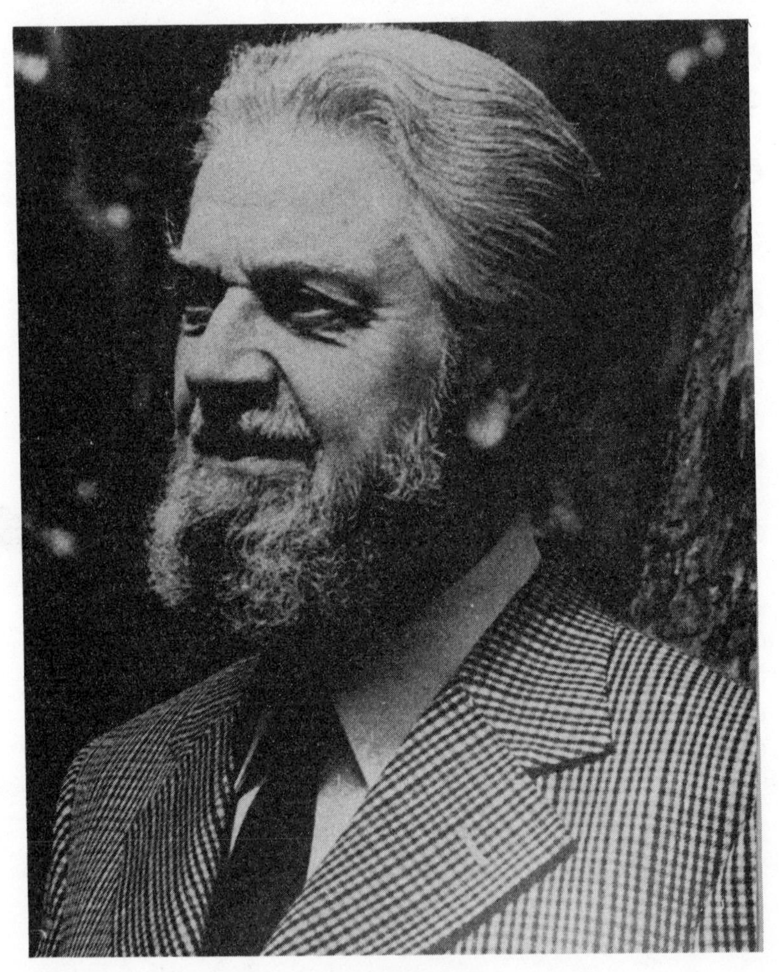

Leslie Sheppard

Leslie Sheppard

Leslie had his first book published by W. Foulshams in 1935 and for nearly half a century was a Violin Expert of International repute. During his business life he wrote hundreds of articles and also had a number of books published, mainly connected with music and musicians.

He received the Eugene Ysaye Medal & Diploma of Honour in Brussels in 1977 for his literary work connected with this famous Belgian Violinist.

Tinnitus and hearing loss caused him to retire in 1983. Over the past ten years he has devoted much of his time and energy to researching and writing on tinnitus. Numerous radio talks and a TV appearance have helped to raise awareness about this poorly understood condition. Currently a number of his articles appear in Journals produced by International Tinnitus Associations. His previous book on Tinnitus "Tinnitus – Learning to live with it" (Ashgrove Press) has gone into two editions and sold in both Britain and America.

This work is the outcome of the close mutual interest in Tinnitus that exists between father and son. Dr Clive Sheppard, a General Practitioner, writes in several medical publications.

Since 1988 Leslie has been Chairman of the Norfolk Tinnitus Society, an Independent Tinnitus Self-Help Group which is one of the largest and most active such Groups in the country.

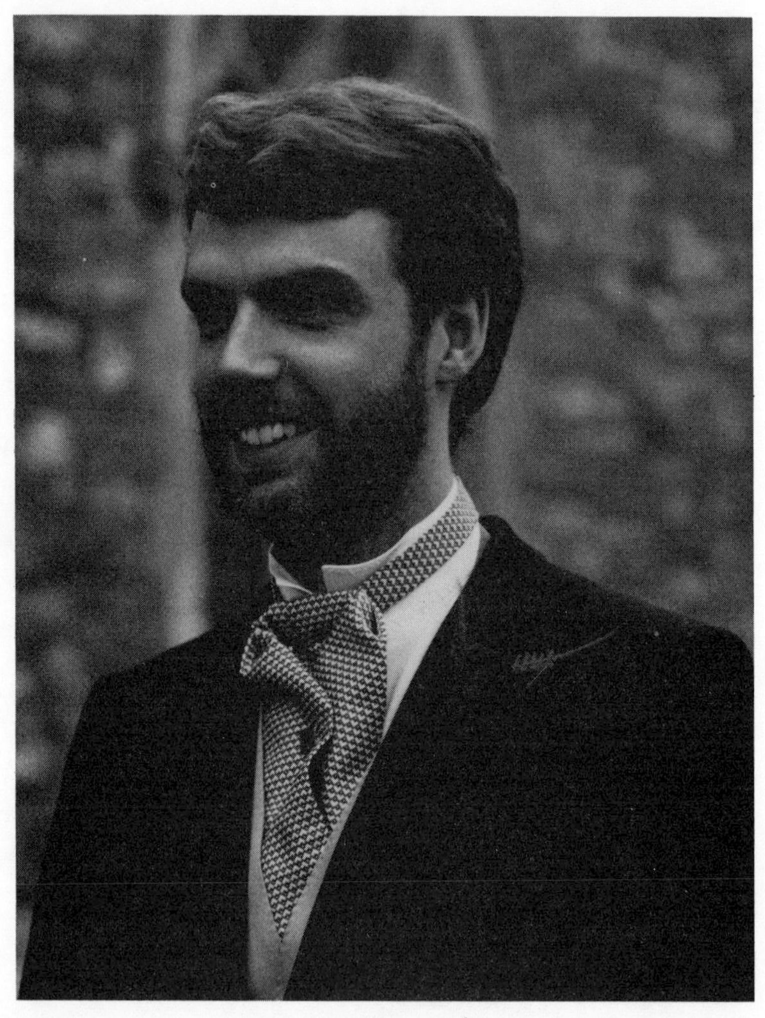

Dr Clive Sheppard

Acknowledgements

This book is the outcome of some ten years of research and study and I regret the sources of information are far too numerous for me to nominate.

I wish to express my most sincere thanks to all Members of the Norfolk Tinnitus Society to which currently over five hundred people with Tinnitus have joined. My close involvement with these dear people has given me the necessary stimulus to complete this book.

I also wish to thank my son Clive for his recommendations and careful editing of the text, and to thank my dear wife Peggy for her encouragement, many suggestions and careful checking of the proofs.

Leslie Sheppard

This book is dedicated to Peggy

Chapter One

The Historical Background of Tinnitus

Quite frankly, until it hit me, I had never heard of Tinnitus, and in fact actually wondered if perhaps it was some new condition brought about by modern living. Later, in my efforts to research the historical background I was amazed to discover that it had in fact been around a very long time, in fact at least before 3000 BC.

Way back in early times any such condition as this would have been thought to be caused by either Gods or Evil Spirits being displeased over something or other. And there would have been far more myth than medicine in the ministrations of the so-called physicians of the day.

For some 1500 years of man's history, medical progress was retarded by what is known as the Humoral Theory in which every ill that befell us was attributed to one of the four humours (or liquids) of the body. And with this muddled thinking when even the 'Doctors' of the day were unable to agree among themselves, it is easy to understand just why the common man still clung to his ancient beliefs and superstitions – after all . . . better the Devil you know . . .

It has only been during the last 300 years or so that healing first began to enter the realms of reality with the realisation at long last that most illnesses have a biological cause. Curiously, this was a mere rebirth of the very theory of Hippocrates who lived as far back as 400 BC.

In an early Egyptian papyrus, thought to date from around 2500 BC a likely reference to tinnitus appears in one section giving instruction for the treatment of a 'bewitched ear'. These early remedies mainly advocated the insertion of various potions into the ear or the fumigation of the ears by smoke from the burning of such things as the skins of non-poisonous snakes.

A much later Egyptian papyrus reported to date from around the 6th century AD specifically mentions 'noises in the ears' which can only indicate Tinnitus, and dating back to the seventh century AD the Assyrians have left us various obvious references to Tinnitus and it would appear that their so called 'treatments' of the condition varied according to the sounds that the sufferer reported hearing. Some of these sounds were regarded as requiring treatment by incantation, whilst others demand purgatives or such treatment as wool soaked in some weird concoction and placed in the offending ear or ears. Probably the main beneficial effects that these things had on the sufferer was that at least the affliction was recognised and something was being done to attempt to relieve it.

A great many early theories regarding Tinnitus existed. For example it was thought that it was caused by air in the ear being trapped and having no outlet. This is a very understandable explanation for those that suffered from the 'shooshing' type of Tinnitus.

In the late 16th century the medical profession favoured a popular form of treatment by the removal of a piece of the skull from the temporal lobe, but alas many of the early attempts at this sort of treatment proved fatal and it was soon dropped.

But the idea that Tinnitus was caused by trapped air was still prevalent in the 16th century when the various sounds that sufferers reported were thought to be entirely due to the differing speed at which this trapped air was escaping, and this idea of trapped air was also behind the earlier efforts of applying actual suction to the ears in an attempt to relieve the situation.

At least from the 17th century onward there appears to be more attention being paid to Tinnitus by the physicians and various reports and papers being written on the subject. Du Verney's work 'Traite de l'organ de l'ouie' published in 1683 was one of the major works of the time and included a section on Tinnitus although admittedly inclining more toward the possibility of brain and ear disease being the cause of the condition.

A work by Wepfer published in 1727 suggested that Tinnitus could be alleviated by loud noises. From the earliest part of the 18th century we find considerable attention being placed on the possibility of Tinnitus being caused by an obstruction in the

Eustachian tube; (the tube which allows air to pass into the middle ear so that the air pressure is kept even on both sides of the ear drum). It being felt that any obstruction here would cause a shortage of air in the middle ear and this resulted in Tinnitus.

The whole of the 19th century saw little real advancement in the treatment of Tinnitus, although certainly there were two fairly important works written on the subject – one by Itard in 1821 and another by MacNaughton-Jones in 1891. And throughout the whole of this century there seems to have been very little progress made toward efforts to relieve Tinnitus. The application of leeches to the legs or to the jugular vein with ice cold douches to the head was advocated, although it was fully realised that such efforts could give but short temporary relief if anything at all.

Some quite primitive suggestions for masking were in vogue, such as a roaring wood fire in the bedroom for murmuring Tinnitus; a damp wood fire for whistling Tinnitus; the fixing of some contrivance for water to drip into a copper pan for ringing Tinnitus; or a noisy spring-driven motor adapted to a mechanised organ for machine-like Tinnitus. Indeed the whole of that century gave us no real development in the management of Tinnitus apart from certain drugs – all of which were discovered to be totally useless.

Attempts at alleviation by static electricity had first been introduced as far back as 1749, and again by Brenner in 1868 who endeavoured to take this treatment a stage further but without success. Later MacNaughton-Jones endeavoured to introduce more advanced electrotherapy for Tinnitus but the result was found to be most disappointing. It was he who advocated percussive massage which he said he found had some effect in certain cases, but all this was very soon dropped.

Two factors occur to me. Firstly, perhaps the percentage of people suffering from tinnitus in those times was much less than in the present day. For in the 17th to 19th centuries the average life-span was nowhere near what it is today. Since the prime cause of tinnitus in the elderly lies in the degeneration of the tiny hair cells of hearing through age, perhaps this would explain it.

Secondly there could well have been an additional reason, for if one complained of 'noises in the head' in those unenlightened times one stood an excellent chance of being regarded as mad, and possibly clapped into an asylum. And a still further fear from presenting one's problem to a physician must surely have arisen from the knowledge of some of the so-called 'remedies'.

There existed however one escape route for sufferers from tinnitus and this lay in the Quack 'Doctors' who flourished from the 17th century onwards, for by reason of their 'cure-all' and all-embracing claims for various potions they could easily be approached with no questions asked. It is here that we can find numerous records of claims for the relief of tinnitus although of course this term was unknown at the time and was referred to by many other quaint names.

The name 'Quack' comes from the astringent voices with which those old salesmen of so-called 'remedies' proclaimed their wares. What is particularly interesting to us is not only the fact that so many included references to tinnitus within the many ills they claimed to cure, but that these people existed and prospered in the community for something like 300 years. There are indeed several famous firms who are household names today whose ancestors go back to the families of some of these people.

The Quacks appear to have surfaced after the death of Oliver Cromwell in 1658; a time of considerable political laxity when hundreds of English Quacks who had for years been operating under cover came out into the open. They were joined by hundreds more from Scotland and Ireland and it was soon not unusual to find as many as a dozen or even more at any village fair or market. They were greatly encouraged by the gullibility of the general public and also by the ease with which licences to operate were granted by the Bishops – perhaps by the crossing of the holy palm with silver?

The impudence and audacity with which these itinerant impostors advertised their wares was truly amazing, and many of them as if not content with the multitude of complaints already waiting to be cured invented diseases, conditions and complaints of their own. For example one 17th century booklet still in existence undertakes to cure among other things, such ills as 'The Glimming of the Glizzard' – 'The Quavering of the Kidneys' and 'The Wambling Trot'.

There exist some amazing accounts of these people, many of whom amassed considerable fortunes. They were of course mere charlatans and by the time the gullible purchaser discovered a remedy to be useless, they were miles away in some other town or village plying their trade.

The largest quack fortunes of all were made in America during the last century. The usual method there was through the establishment of what was called 'The Medical Institutes' which were purely commercial concerns. These had Medical Museums attached to them displaying waxwork figures of people purported to be showing the effects of various serious diseases. The effects were so nauseating that many of the visitors fell ill, and of course this was the whole idea. Attendants known as 'floor men' were constantly on hand to come forward and offer sympathy and advice, soon convincing the victims that they were showing obvious signs of some disease or other and suggested they should have a free consultation with the 'Eminent Specialist' upstairs. Once there within the spider's web it was but a matter of minutes before the diagnosis was confirmed, but hope was held out if the victims were willing to sign up for a full course of treatment!

Here then is our picture of the medical scene of the past, and in such times let us spare a thought for those with tinnitus in those days. They were truly in an invidious position. To go to any physician for help with 'noises in the head' would mean there was a very fair chance of ending up in the local asylum or other institution. The only answer was therefore identical with so much medical advice given today – 'learn to live with it'. Thus can we appreciate just why the false promises of the Quacks was so irresistible, for the sufferer was then in a non-threatening situation. The remedy which was purported to cure so many ills without actually specifying the ill itself meant that the seller was never aware of the buyer's problem in any case, and if the potion did no good the buyer was not in any position to complain.

These poor people were thus entirely in the hands of these charlatans, who would return time and time again offering new and all-embracing 'remedies' and in latter years these actually did include cures for 'jingling in the ears' – 'caterwauling eardrums' – 'bells in the head' and any other designations of tinnitus that were popular at the time.

Chapter Two

Some Facts About Tinnitus

The latin word 'tinnire' means to ring as one would ring a bell, and it is from this that the word Tinnitus derives. It is best described as referring to a noise or noises heard by a person but has no environmental source that can be objectively verified.

The noises heard vary considerably and the most usual are described as humming, buzzing, ringing or shooshing like a sea shell held to the ear. Others talk of shrieking, hissing, clicking, chirping or of a low throbbing hum. Another form is the sound of the heart-beat, this is known as pulsatile Tinnitus. I feel sure that many with Tinnitus will find themselves identifying with one or other of these descriptions, with others able to add to them.

It must at the outset be emphasised that Tinnitus is a symptom of auditory dysfunction or degeneration and is not a disease in itself. Unfortunately, despite considerable research, as things stand at the moment there is no known general cure and in this one can only feel genuinely sorry for General Practitioners, ENT Consultants etc. who when presented with the problem by their patients have to tell them that they must 'learn to live with it' for in this regard the whole medical profession must feel inadequate and helpless. Many GP's may well try to help by prescribing some drug (usually an antidepressant) but so often by reason of the side effects these do little to actually help. In fact they can all too easily exacerbate this very devious condition.

Wherever possible however, it is always prudent and advisable for anyone with Tinnitus to undergo a full auditory examination if only to prove that nothing can be done medically by way of help.

Many people experiencing Tinnitus for the first time become extremely anxious, thinking they have perhaps a cerebral tumour. So many at this stage become suicidal, feeling that they can no longer live with this torment day and night. It is known that there are many actual suicides due to Tinnitus, but of course coroners' reports nearly always refer to 'depressive illness' or some such term. It is a great pity for the sake of publicising the dangers of Tinnitus that the truth is not told.

Tinnitus causes considerable depression in most sufferers, especially in the early stages. It is also extremely debilitating and can cause considerable irritability to the detriment of relationships, together with a feeling of inadequateness and helplessness.

An interesting analysis of the ages of Tinnitus patients who were attending a large Tinnitus Clinic for the first time some 20 years ago is given below:

	Age	*No of cases*
FEMALES	25	8
	33	12
	45	14
	55*	33*
	65	20
	84	1
MALE	5	1
	15	2
	24	11
	33	10
	44	17
	55*	22*
	62	9
	92	1

* This increase with both sexes in middle age was thought to be possibly due to the acoustic trauma of the war years.

If the Tinnitus is the result of some underlying ear problem or some other physical condition it is sometimes possible for the Tinnitus to be relieved depending on the condition. If it is due to correctable ear disease it may well be possible to have this attended to and so obtain relief. Or if sufferers are found to be on drugs or medications which either produce or aggravate Tinnitus then the sufferer can be weaned off such medications as necessary.

In all these instances there is some hope of alleviation of the

Tinnitus even to the point of cure, but alas such cases are lamentably few and far between.

All tinnitus sufferers should be cautioned to avoid excessive noise and those in occupations with a high noise level are advised most strongly to use adequate ear protection. It is however unfortunate that with a number of people with this condition the reduction in the strength of the environmental noise when wearing ear defenders only tends to heighten the awareness of their own Tinnitus. Yet if they totally reject the use of such defenders or other protective devices on the basis that occlusion makes their Tinnitus more perceptible, they must be made fully aware of the possible consequences both as regards further loss of hearing and increased Tinnitus.

However, many people work in noisy environments in which it is vital that they are able to hear the sound of warnings or signals; similarly others, such as singers and musicians of all kinds, orchestral conductors and so on must at all times be able to hear the music they are producing. Here the suggestion has been made that one protective device is used and moved from ear to ear every hour or so, but this seems a poor partial solution indeed.

It is always somewhat surprising that the symptom of Tinnitus can prove to be such a debilitating problem. Fear – stress – depression and insomnia resulting from the condition all have their part to play in this, and any degree of help in alleviating these other factors can help tremendously. The claustrophobic effect of hearing constant hissing, moaning, shushing, chirping, roaring, humming and all the other horrendous sounds that Tinnitus can bring, create considerable debilitation which can become a vicious circle causing even greater tension in the auditory system.

The actual site of Tinnitus is also a problem, for it can arise from so many locations in the auditory chain . . . the middle ear . . . the cochlea . . . or the various nerves and neurological areas, and in some cases it does not even arise in the hearing mechanism at all.

At one time it was thought that sectioning the auditory nerve was a cure. This was given considerable publicity, but such surgery does not work in those cases where the Tinnitus originates from the brain itself and the success rate was dismally low. It also resulted in complete deafness in the ear that was operated on.

Other surgical attempts were labyrinthectomy (the surgical removal of part or the whole of the membraneous labyrinth in the inner ear), and fenestration (the creation of an opening in the inner ear for the relief of deafness in otosclerosis which is a condition of new bone formation usually affecting the labyrinth) but neither of these, nor other surgical attempts have been very successful, often making matters far worse for the patients involved.

Another area of research has been that of electrical stimulation for long term relief of Tinnitus, but alas again results are somewhat disappointing.

The reassurance obtained by a sufferer following the ruling out of any serious disease and the assurance that the Tinnitus is not harmful, certainly relieves some of the hitherto resulting stress, but the noises still remain of course, and sufferers should know that this can be made all the worse when they allow themselves to become tense, worried or tired. Those situations likely to cause them such exacerbation should therefore be avoided as far as possible, although as we are all aware it is very difficult to do this in modern life. Far too many people with Tinnitus avoid socialising due to their feelings of insecurity stemming from hearing loss or the inability to hear in a crowded room. This is a great pity, because it would be preferable for them to increase their social or physical activities both of which could form a distraction from their Tinnitus.

So often in their anguish Tinnitus sufferers will threaten suicide – this is a matter which even hinted at needs immediate counselling. It should be discussed at once and never ignored. The person's GP should be notified at once of any threat of suicide. Any such apparent preparation should also be reported at once – such as acquiring a gun, saving drugs or even making a will.

It is generally agreed that alcohol in any form can affect Tinnitus quite badly, and this is very evident after excessive use. It is thought to be due to the disturbance of blood flow. Some people are quite adamant that alcohol relieves their Tinnitus, but one can only assume that this is due mainly to the fact that it causes them to temporarily relax, probably paying for this slight relief later on.

Caffeine is a substance known to be bad for anyone with Tinnitus. This means that tea, coffee, chocolate, cocoa and Cola drinks all of which contain considerable caffeine, should be taken at least cautiously. It is best for anyone with Tinnitus to use decaffeinated tea and coffee wherever possible. Caffeine is also present in numerous other things that we buy – look at the labels.

Additionally, our hearing mechanism is one of the most sensitive parts of our body and Tinnitus can often be tracked down to one of the many side effects of certain synthetic drugs and antibiotics.

Pulsatile Tinnitus is a fairly rare symptom. This type asserts itself by a regular pulsating noise in the head or ears most usually in precise rhythm with the heart beat.

Some forms of the disorder can be controlled by embolism (the partial blocking of a blood vessel etc) but the vast majority of cases seem to be connected with the transmission of energy waves from the vessels around the brain through the cochlear aquaduct. Some patients have been fitted with a special 'balloon' catheter inside a blood vessel. By blowing up the balloon, blood flow is reduced and so effects of change in circulation on the tinnitus can be assessed.

Tinnitus is certainly devious, to say the least. It can appear to be coming from various parts of the head or even outside the head. It may occur in only one ear; it can occur in both ears; there can be the same sound in both ears or a differing sound in each ear. The noise may even move around from ear to ear. With some people it can disappear altogether for certain periods; very rarely it can even disappear completely, all for no obvious reason. It can remain at constant volume or it can change in its intensity from time to time. But with most people Tinnitus occurs in either the same ear or both ears constantly, with sound and volume fairly level throughout.

Although there are several theories as to the specific mechanism causing Tinnitus this is not really yet fully understood. At present there appear to be two opposing theories.

One theory is that Tinnitus is due to the spontaneous firing of auditory nerve fibres. The slower the discharge rate, the less the severity of the Tinnitus. This has been described by one expert as 'an itch in the hair cells of the cochlea'.

Another theory – that of Kiang, Moxon and Levine is entirely different to this, stating that . . . . "Tinnitus is something that is not actually there" The theory is that certain hair cells of the cochlea have been destroyed for one reason or another and the result is that this causes a sensation of sound such as the sensation experienced by amputees over 'phantom limbs'.

Although both theories are connected with the action or otherwise of nerve cells, both fail in several ways to explain all the variations of tinnitus that plague sufferers.

In a very few special cases surgery *has* been successful in curing it, but most attempts have failed and in many cases have even exacerbated the condition rather than alleviated it.

Chapter Three
Tinnitus Problems

The Institute of Hearing Research issued a postal Questionnaire some years ago taking names at random from the Electoral Registers of four fairly large towns in Great Britain. This requested a self-reported hearing state from the recipients under such headings as:

No complaint?
Some Hearing Loss?
Both Hearing Loss & Tinnitus?
Age?
Gender?
Noise Exposure at work?
Do you possess a Hearing Aid?

About fifty per cent of those who replied accepted the invitation to attend the Hearing Clinic in their respective town and a follow-up of a home visit which included simple audiometry.

Those people who reported having Tinnitus only after exposure to loud sounds such as discos, shooting, or loud noise at work, and only those reporting Tinnitus of some duration were included in this Survey.

The Survey indicated that 15½% of the population of Southampton, and 18½% of the city of Glasgow had Tinnitus of extended duration. In each case 5% of those with Tinnitus reported difficulty in getting to sleep due to the symptom. Those reporting very severe Tinnitus, sufficient to seriously affect the quality of their lives was at the ratio of one in every two hundred of the population.

The report of the Office of Population Censuses & Surveys of 1983 states, regarding the prevalence of Tinnitus at that time:

'As to the prevalence of Tinnitus in adults – that is from the age of 17 and over,about 22% of those interviewed said that they had heard noises in their head and ears such as ringing or hunger, thirst or pain can find their way into the dream sequence.

Experts inform us that it has been established beyond any doubt that dreaming is essential to good health, and modern research confirms that sleep is most important, as loss of sleep can impair both brain function and concentration. After only 48 hours without sleep the body begins to generate a stress substance very similar to LSD.

Without doubt a good sleep regenerates the body, repairs damaged tissues and cells and strengthens the immune system as well as making one feel mentally relaxed.

Difficulty in sleeping is said to affect one in five of us at some stage of our lives. If you suffer from insomnia it is important for you to look for possible causes apart from the actual noises of Tinnitus. Look for other stress factors and do remember that all sleeping tablets mar normal sleep and affect the degree to which you dream.

The taking of sleeping pills is something of a modern mania. In Britain alone it is estimated that over 300 million sleeping pills are prescribed every year. There are five different types of sleeping drugs:

The Benzodiazepines comprise the most commonly used class. The Barbiturates are now rarely used because of the risks of dependence, and the danger of toxicity in overdosage.

The Non-Barbiturate sleeping drugs were originally developed as safer alternatives to Barbiturates and there are new drugs in this category that are said to have advantages over the Benzodiazepines but these are still under study.

The Antihistamines are used to treat allergic symptoms such as connected with animal fur, house dust, pollen and so on. They can cause drowsiness and are sometimes used in Insomnia in elderly people and children.

Some Antidepressant drugs used in treating underlying depressive illness help to promote sleep in depressed people. These drugs can take between six and eight weeks before a patient feels the full effect and during that time certain side effects may be experienced which often cause patients to discontinue the medication.

Because the sleep induced by drugs is not the same as normal sleep, many feel that they do not find themselves so well rested as in a night of normal sleep. This is caused by suppressed brain activity and also because such drugs suppress that stage of sleep in which we dream, and dream sleep and non dream sleep are both essential components for a proper night's rest in order to maintain good health.

It must be pointed out that most sleeping drugs apart from the anti-histamines can produce both psychological and physical dependence when taken regularly for more than a few weeks, and especially if taken in larger than normal doses.

If these drugs are withdrawn abruptly, sleeplessness, anxiety, fits and hallucinations can arise. Nightmares and vivid dreams can occur as the amount of time in dream sleep increases to make up for what has been lost during the medication.

The usual medical aids for insomnia are hypnotic drugs. Anaesthetics used in surgery and hypnotic drugs are very closely related. They induce a coma caused by the poisoning of the brain cells. The patient wakes eventually when the body has eliminated the poison. In this lies the danger of taking sleeping pills over the prescribed dosage. The other risk of taking sleeping pills is that over a long period there can be a temptation to exceed the stated dose since their effect diminishes over a few weeks.

If the difficulty in sleeping is so great that one really must use drugs, then it is best to try to get your doctor to prescribe different drugs which are appropriate to your case, and experiment with these over a few days. A drug that agrees with one person does not necessarily agree with another.

It is only when one is fully justified in resorting to drugs for sleep, such as when Insomnia has proved incurable, that one should take such drugs. In such cases as this these drugs can certainly help re-establish your normal sleep routine and are a useful method of regaining normal sleep patterns again, but the dangers mentioned still apply.

In general it is far better to learn and practice a personal relaxation technique than to rely on drug treatments for insomnia unless that insomnia is due to underlying depression.

We have now covered some of the elements of sleep itself. Now let us face the problem of a person with Tinnitus and the additional burden of Insomnia with which to cope.

Anything which soothes and relaxes such as a hot drink can

buzzing sounds. Subsequent questions established that in about one third of these informants the noises were brought on only by an external stimulus such as loud noise, water getting into the ears, or cold or catarrh. But 2% of the population said they were bothered a great deal by their Tinnitus.'

Some International Surveys give estimates of Tinnitus prevalence in the populations of modern industrialised countries of between 35% and 45% of adults experiencing Tinnitus at some time or other, with even the short term sufferers reporting that it is a considerable nuisance to them.

At least 8% appear to experience Tinnitus to a severity which interferes with their getting to sleep, and this figure alone suggests that around four million adults in the United Kingdom are thus affected. Also with the incidence of one in every 200 of the population suffering from very severe Tinnitus in the United Kingdom, although this sounds a small proportion, in total it amounts to some 200,000 sufferers.

There is a trend toward higher prevalence of Tinnitus in women than in men. This was indicated in a population study in Britain during 1981 and another study in the USA where 30% of males reported Tinnitus compared to 35% of females.

However, some experts point to the statistics of the extended life-span of women to that of men, and are inclined to feel that this might bring the incidence of male to female ratio to a more even match.

In reports from such areas as Cardiff, Glasgow, Nottingham and Southampton, the prevalence of Tinnitus causing severe effect on the ability to lead a normal life, show no differences in percentages.

One interesting feature arising from all these reports is the indication that Tinnitus occurs more frequently in the left ear than the right. There have been various suppositions put forward as reasons for this, but few hold water.

The really interesting outcome from these various surveys so far as those with Tinnitus are concerned, comes from the indication that although so many have been advised to 'Learn to Live with it' – a remark which seems so very harsh at the outset, one does in some way become more accustomed to the noises when experienced over a considerable period (described by the medical profession as 'a tending towards habituation').

It is certainly the opinion of those who have lived for some time with Tinnitus of a level intensity that it is not now as disturbing or seemingly loud as it was at the outset. However, I agree this is small consolation.

When asked to list the main difficulties pertaining to Tinnitus many people will say that it is the way in which it interferes with their understanding of speech. This is rather doubtful since one could almost say that many – almost the majority – of people with Tinnitus also have a certain degree of hearing loss and this would surely be the main cause of this particular difficulty – not the Tinnitus. There are also other features such as the feeling of insecurity plus perhaps a little irritability inclining one not to take the trouble to listen too intently, or even the distraction to concentration brought on by the tinnitus noise itself.

The localization of sounds (i.e. not being able to tell from which direction a sound is coming) is also very difficult for anyone with hearing loss markedly in one ear, for it is the fact that we have two ears that enables us to localize the direction of sounds.

Certainly there are some difficulties attributable to Tinnitus itself, such as insomnia, the withdrawal from and avoidance of company and problems with relationships within the family circle. Some of the difficulties can also affect one's general health. Frequent headaches are one feature as is a feeling of giddiness and imbalance. Tinnitus can also often cause a certain degree of ill-health in some people, especially those who are highly strung, and thus find its persistence more debilitating than others. Tiredness is another feature and this can often be made even worse by a person attempting to 'keep busy' as an antidote to the noises in their head.

Add to these things those associated symptoms of the condition which complete a vicious circle of exacerbation such as despair, frustration, depression, annoyance, irritation, inability to concentrate, inability to relax properly, the feeling of insecurity, worry, fear and suicidal tendencies, and we are beginning to complete the picture of the tinnitus sufferer and to better understand their world.

These are only some of the great diversity of problems that beset one when experiencing really severe Tinnitus, for nothing has yet been said of the spoiling of the quality of life by such things as not being able to enjoy listening to music or watching television. Many find it additionally irritating by reason of the fact that they are not able to explain exactly what the noise IS that they are experiencing constantly in their head or ears. And as we are all aware it is extremely difficult for those without Tinnitus to really appreciate just what devastating proportions the symptom can sometimes assume.

Against all this however, there are people with Tinnitus in a fairly mild form who are not sufficiently troubled to even seek relief, and in fact do nothing about it. Though alas there is often all too little that CAN be done.

There are also two other distinct categories. Some seek noisy surroundings to offset the effects of the noise of their Tinnitus, whilst others avoid noisy situations like the plague. This is especially true of those who experience Recruitment.

There are several difficulties which those with severe Tinnitus share equally with hearing-impaired or deaf people. Both know full well that their problem makes life harder for them by difficulty in listening to speech ... in other words essential communication ... and which often makes them feel stupid before others. Add to this the difficulty of hearing ordinary environmental sounds plus the inability to localize sound, and it is small wonder that both suffer from a certain sense of loneliness, insecurity and depression, plus additional difficulties if at work.

Yet strangely, in various researches into the subject, each group regard the importance of such difficulties in their lives quite differently. The hearing-impaired section seem to regard problems associated with work as being twice as important to them as do those with Tinnitus. This may well be through those in the former group experiencing more problems in communication.

The possible dramatic consequences of Tinnitus were well illustrated in a research programme of 50 people with Tinnitus taken at random at one certain clinic, among which no less than 5 reported that they had at some time or times seriously considered suicide. In such cases as this very careful counselling is required immediately, together with the provision of expert information followed by a discussion of the possible treatments available with emphasis laid on all the emotional problems related to the condition, and advice given on how one can try to help oneself to cope in this situation.

It is somewhat difficult to disentangle the many problems that have been mentioned in order to state that this or that has affected a person in a certain way, for there is much correlation between them. Thus in counselling it is essential that all the problems existing should be taken into consideration, and not just one problem taken in isolation.

The manifold problems which Tinnitus can bring are not always easily apparent on the surface. A fair number of those with Tinnitus find it overwhelming by reason of the fact that they are unable to cope with it emotionally. I have just read of one case in which Tinnitus has caused divorce and this is by no means an isolated instance.

This lady was divorced at the age of thirty-six. Her Tinnitus had started some fifteen years before. She has two children – both at school. Before Tinnitus struck her the marriage was perfectly happy and secure, but gradually her condition began to affect and disrupt not only their family life but the sexual relationship with her husband. She came to a point where she found it impossible to even join her family in sitting and watching the television, since any loud sounds affected her badly (recruitment). She suffered insomnia in consequence of her Tinnitus and became reluctant to join the rest of the family on any outings, she became depressed and morose to an extent that others were inclined to avoid her company.

Her Tinnitus caused her to sleep badly and made her extremely reluctant to go to bed at night until very late – generally quite some hours after her husband had retired. This reluctance not only frustrated her spouse but doubtless he misinterpreted the reason. Coupled with other matters all this so badly affected their sexual relationship that they eventually mutually agreed to separate, and were divorced a year or so later. There is no doubt whatever that Tinnitus was the sole cause of the break-up of this particular marriage and I am aware of other instances.

Another case of the effects of Tinnitus upon a person is that of a sixty-five year old widow who has had Tinnitus for only three years. In this instance it caused a complete change of personality in quite a short space of time.

Previously she had led a very active life, belonged to several clubs and to the WI, and would regularly baby-sit for either of her married daughters both of whom lived nearby. Now gradually since the onset of her Tinnitus she hardly goes out at all; she has become unkempt in her appearance having 'let herself go'. She never visits either of her daughters, being only too aware that she is bad company and an unhappy influence. Her general health has deteriorated badly, and since she is now experiencing attacks of vertigo refuses to use her cooker as she is afraid of falling on it following several near misses. She thus exists mainly on breakfast cereals and sandwiches. Tinnitus is solely responsible for bringing this previously normal and happy person to this sorry state.

Due to ageing a great number of elderly people suffer from severe and intractable Tinnitus. The vicious circle produced results in their finding it intolerable when they become depressed, tired or under stress. So many of these people live alone which makes their position even worse, for to be able to talk about one's difficulties is not only helpful but additionally therapeutic. On top of this they are so often retired and therefore have much time on their hands with little to occupy them. They have few activities outside the home and are inclined to be introspective regarding their general health.

Such people usually do not sleep well or make certain that they have proper meals and they may become easily depressed and debilitated.

Chapter Four

Severity and Age Factors

An important investigation into the severity of Tinnitus was undertaken in Portland, Oregon, from over 1800 patients attending a Tinnitus Clinic there. These patients were asked to rate their tinnitus on a scale comparison from 1 to 10 with 'mild tinnitus' being in the region of 1 to 2.

Unfortunately for a great number of reasons an accurate assessment of tinnitus is extremely difficult. Far too many people are inclined to equate loudness with severity, yet in others the severity itself has no relation to loudness but is judged more on how personally disturbing the noises are.

This became apparent from the information gained from nearly two thousand patients who had been at the Tinnitus Clinic of the Oregon Health Sciences University over a six year period.

The method involved required each to complete a brief questionnaire followed by an audiological examination, plus a number of tinnitus tests including the possibility of masking.

Each patient was asked how long they had suffered from tinnitus, their past otologic history and general medical history, together with any information regarding the knowledge of noise exposure and so on. This was followed by each patient estimating the severity of their tinnitus on the horizonal scale previously mentioned. Most were able to do this but some indicated more than one degree of severity whilst others were unable to give any such indication at all.

Then followed an attempt to determine the pitch or frequency of a sound which appeared to the patient to best match the pitch of his tinnitus. This was followed by attempting to determine the loudness level and determination of the sensation level and an attempt to discover the best external sound to mask the tinnitus. Then followed a test of residual inhibition [this is when the tinnitus remains temporarily quiet following the cessation of the masking effect.]

It was found that with those with moderate hearing loss and the pitch of their tinnitus not above from 3 to 4 kHz a hearing aid or aids was all that was required. In others, effective masking of the tinnitus was found possible with either a usual tinnitus masker or a combination masker/hearing aid. However, in some patients it was impossible to mask the tinnitus despite all attempts.

From computerized statistics the characteristics of all these patients was summarized as follows. There were 1806 patients involved, 69% were male and 31% female. These percentages are somewhat strange since in Great Britain the incidence is very much biased toward the female population.

Age distribution was	up to 20	3%
	21 to 30	6%
	31 to 40	13%
	41 to 50	17%
	51 to 60	28%
	61 to 70	23%
	71 & over	10%

The patients involved in this investigation came from all over the United States and Canada, including a number from other countries. The majority came from the Pacific NW.

With regard to the statements which now follow, it must be pointed out that the number of patients can be variable in each particular. This arises from sample sizes differing either by reason of some of the sufferers being unable to perform certain tests say from physical incapacity or extreme hearing loss, or the omission of some answers to the questionnaire. Also those patients who gave more than one severity level due to fluctuating tinnitus were omitted completely.

However, 1361 patients gave precise answers, and data on the loudness of their tinnitus was obtained from some 50% of these. The highest severity ratings were between 7 & 8 on the scale. The sensation levels in dB given by 584 patients matching tinnitus loudness to external sounds showed that the large majority were at 0–3 dB. Hardly any correlation was found between the loudness and the severity of this tinnitus.

It is felt that the method of matching loudness of tinnitus may well be somewhat imperfect, for matching is mostly performed with the same frequency as that of the tinnitus. However, this frequency can often be at the very spot in the hearing spectrum at which the greatest loss can be found, and therefore loudness recruitment could result in a completely inaccurate assessment. With extra increase in the loudness, the sensation levels could well represent large increases in the perceived loudness thus causing the measurements to be deceptively low. Such conditions can cause the loudness obtained to be as much as 20 dB higher than indicated at tinnitus frequency.

In analysing the individual answers to the questionnaire relating to severity and loudness there was no correlation between patients' ratings of these two features. For example, in three cases of patients giving a severity level of 7 one described the loudness level as being 'the level of a diesel truck motor'; another as 'the loudness of an electric fan'; and a third as 'the loudness of a police siren'.

In this particular test some unreliability was also reported since some patients found it necessary to place their degree of loudness or severity mid-way between the stated degrees of intensity on the chart.

An interesting feature of this test was that all taking part were asked to describe in some detail precisely what sounds they were actually hearing, The answers were 'hissing' – 'the sound of crickets' – 'ocean roar' – 'steam whistle' etc. However, quite a number of patients reported more than one particular sound in their tinnitus [i.e. complex sounds]. Those who reported only one sound numbered 856; 383 spoke of two sounds; 161 of three sounds; 76 of four different sounds; and 28 of five sounds. The conclusion was also drawn that those who reported only one or two sounds had a much lower severity rating than those reporting four or five sounds.

In around 70% of these patients it was found that their tinnitus could be masked by ear level equipment such as tinnitus maskers, combination instruments (masker plus a hearing aid) and with some just a hearing aid alone. Those patients gaining the most relief from masking were also those who reported that they were able to gain some relief from ambient environmental noise.

The majority of the patients in whom the tinnitus could not be masked were those who reported the higher severity ratings, and this indicated that there must be some relationship existing between severity and successful masking.

As to severity, there were no particular age-related trends nor any great differences between male and female as regards severity.

A study was made on the information gained concerning past medical history and noise exposure history – 34% had received head injury at some time during their lives. Those who had experienced ear infection or disease numbered 23% and 69% had been exposed to loud noise at some time or other. It was found that there was no difference whatever in regard to severity ratings for either of these groups.

As to the medical condition of the patients tested, 21% had allergy problems; 16% reported hypertension, 4% had diabetes and 2% reported cardiovascular disease. Only 1% reported arthritis, thyroid disfunction, sinusitis, headache or migraine, and none of these conditions connected with either high or low severity ratings.

Among the behavioural indications of this test insomnia and general sleep-disturbance was the general problem experienced by patients. Many reported problems of concentration, maintenance of normal social relationships with both families, friends and workmates, and interference with the ability to properly relax.

The tests had certainly shown that it would be helpful to investigate the matter of the severity of tinnitus and find ways and means of measuring this more accurately. It was felt that the measurements of loudness using a comparison noise need to take into account the ever-present possibility of loudness recruitment within the frequency range covered by the actual pitch of the tinnitus sound. The improvement in loudness evaluation technique would be helpful in evaluating alterations of the severity of the tinnitus [as perceived] caused for example by certain drug therapies. It was also borne in mind that very many patients with only mild tinnitus would not be seeking medical help and would therefore be excluded from the patients who were available for this particular test. A large proportion of those tested had come from doctors' referrals and would therefore have relatively severe tinnitus. This was evident from the very few patients who fell into the lowest category of the severity range when tested.

A very frequent question is "At what age is Tinnitus most likely to start?" This is rather difficult to answer for there are many records of tinnitus affecting people from birth and yet again of commencing near the age of ninety! However, a careful study of all available information seems to point to around the age of 45, but the incidence then rises considerably up to the age of 50 reaching its absolute peak in the 50 to 60 age group. It thus appears that if one is to develop Tinnitus at all it is most likely to start between the ages of 40 to 60.

In reviewing this question it seems likely that there may be several different factors at work in producing the most frequent onset of the symptom of Tinnitus in the 50 to 60 age group, for by this age one has accumulated considerable noise exposure, probably taken a number of drugs that are injurious to the auditory system, plus the additional very strong likelihood of age having caused various degenerative influences on the auditory system.

So far as the matter regarding the influence of drugs is concerned, we must remember that it is around the 40 to 60 age range that most of us develop various aches and pains necessitating a visit to our General Practitioner who may well prescribe a drug. It is of course wise for anyone with hearing problems of any sort, especially Tinnitus, to make this problem known to their doctor at the time of being prescribed any drug.

As to noise exposure, by the time we reach even the age of 40 we have of necessity received considerable exposure to noise, whether this be industrial noise to which we have had to subject ourselves in order to earn a living: accumulated noise exposure received over years of noise hazard from such things as overloud music, discos, hi-fi's and so on, or through loud noises such as sustained in sports – shooting etc.

As to the various additional influences that age can bring we must remember the various other alterations that occur in the inner ear as we grow older. The vibrating basilar membrane of the inner ear becomes thicker and less responsive to external sounds, and the little hair cells so essential to hearing begin to degenerate. Additionally, there may well be less effective blood supply. Impaired hearing known medically as Presbyacusis is described as being a diminution of hearing as age advances. However, this actual process commences as early as the age of 17 when adolescents of that age are unable to hear very high pitched sounds that were perfectly audible to them a few years before. More and more of these high frequencies are lost as age increases until although vowel sounds are heard well, certain consonants are difficult to distinguish, making speech difficult to hear. At this stage such a person is very susceptible to Tinnitus and may well actually have it by then.

But this matter is not quite so clear-cut as it may appear. Whether the onset of Tinnitus actually arises from noise exposure, drug exposure or age is in the majority of cases impossible to judge with any accuracy. Perhaps in certain cases it is a mixture of all three at work together. It has certainly been proved that a passing type of Tinnitus caused by noise exposure may well become regular Tinnitus as late as some twenty years afterwards.

It would be thought that those people who had experienced noise exposure for a considerable period would be more likely to develop Tinnitus earlier than those with a shorter record of such exposure. However research does not bear this out. In a recent project on this very question it was found that in a considerable number of sufferers with the average age of onset around 45 it was found that there was no difference whatever in the number of those who had experienced noise exposure for five years or less, when compared with those who had experienced such exposure for ten years or more. Additionally there appears to be no remarkable difference in the age of onset of Tinnitus through noise exposure between men and women. However it is always said that Tinnitus itself, for whatever reason, is more common in women than men.

Chapter Five

Complementary Medicines in Tinnitus

PART ONE

Complementary Medicine includes all those therapies and approaches to healing that are not covered by orthodox medicine. When attempting to apply any of these to Tinnitus their help in the reduction of the effects of the associated symptoms such as stress, depression, anxiety, lack of concentration, difficulties in relaxing, sleep disorders and the like is usually sought rather than an approach with any expectation of actual cure of the tinnitus itself.

It should be known that some of the Practitioners of Complementary Medicine have had no actual training, whereas others have undergone rigorous full time courses comparable to the undergraduate medical curriculum. There are also now many General Practitioners as well as Consultants who have studied these various therapies.

Most of the Complementary Medicines now have their own central Association and it is best to write here requesting the name and address of your nearest qualified practitioner as a safeguard.

These Complementary Medicines can roughly be divided into four separate groups:

(a) Complete systems of Healing such as Homoeopathy, Chiropractic, Osteopathy, Herbal Medicine & Acupuncture.

(b) Diagnostic methods – Kinesiology – Hair Analysis & Iridology.

(c) Therapeutic methods such as Aromatherapy, Reflexology, and Massage.

(d) Self Help methods such as Meditation, Exercise, Relaxation, Visualisation or Cognitive Therapy.

It will have been noticed that the word 'holistic' is so often used in conjunction with quite a number of Complementary Medicines, and this implies willingness to take into account other factors in the causation of the presented problem.

The major conditions presented to GP's are Depression – Anxiety – Respiratory Disorders – Skin Disease and Pain. In that order. And as many doctors will tell you these will all respond in some degree to several of the approaches made by the appropriate Alternative Medicine. It is not always best for the G.P. to reach for the prescription pad.

The Research Council for Complementary Medicine was established in 1983. However, there are unfortunately many Alternative Practitioners who still lack the time, expertise, or inclination to thoroughly study and evaluate their methods. But the orthodox Medical Profession are willing to work with those Alternative Practitioners who have received a properly constituted training, and whose approaches to treatment have obviously something to offer to their patients. Gradually these people are becoming involved in the whole concept of Health Care and being invited to join the medical profession in their practices and health centres.

The Tinnitus sufferer will obviously select from the wide variety of Alternative Medicines, that which appears to offer the most opportunity for the relief of the associated symptoms of this condition – such as Depression – Anxiety – Sleep Disturbance and so on. To turn to Alternative Medicine for the sole object of avoiding surgery would be a very dangerous and unwise reason for doing so. Reputable Practitioners in the 'alternative field' on discovering that a patient visited them for this reason will always endeavour to help them cope with their fears and persuade them to go back to their doctor.

Any approach that can help in the emotional response of a Tinnitus sufferer can only be helpful. Muscle relaxation certainly has the effect of reducing one's general anxiety state, and thus any alternative medicine that offers this effect is useful. The less anxious one becomes, the less severe the Tinnitus appears to be, for fear and anxiety cause a contraction in the muscles of the neck which result in an alteration in the circulation of the auditory system.

Thus any system of muscle relaxation such as Yoga or Hypnotherapy etc is very helpful for Tinnitus and is usually taken up by sessions with the respective expert followed by the use of special tapes for home use.

Some experts advocate the use of Biofeedback coupled with Relaxation Training. However, much depends on the attitudes of patients to their Tinnitus since many regard the symptom as strictly medical, and if one rejects the idea of any psychological approach, then Biofeedback can be of little use to them. In such cases as this, it is better for patients to practice the skill of relaxation and use it during any particularly bad sessions of Tinnitus.

A BMA report which considered the increase in popularity of alternative medicine particularly laid stress on one particular factor common to many of these therapies, and that was the use of the actual physical contact with a patient plus the 'authoritative attitude' and the 'magical quality' which is attributed to many of these therapies – and possibly to even some of the practitioners!

Most doctors are quite willing to work in conjunction with alternative practitioners in an effort to expand their concept of health care. Any patient desiring to seek help from an alternative medicine should, if only as a matter of courtesy inform their doctor accordingly. In many such cases they will find their GP willing to suggest a reliable local practitioner in that particular sphere.

Over a million people a year seek help from the Alternative Practitioners, and currently there are over 30,000 of these offering their services to the public. On the face of it, it appears somewhat unlikely that any treatments for which literally thousands of people are willing to pay fairly expensive fees should be without some merit. However, in certain sections of the medical profession there has been marked hostility in the past, although the situation is rather different today.

The main objections from the medical profession were based on the fact that a qualified doctor must undergo long and rigorous training with both practical and theoretical examinations, whereas few of the 'fringe medicine' Practitioners had undergone such training in anatomy, physiology and pathology and they objected to diagnosis and treatment being undertaken by such people.

Additionally, orthodox practitioners are of opinion that the causes of all diseases are numerous and that it is not possible for one form of treatment to suffice for a mass of entirely different diseases.

Doctors are further of opinion that whilst the results of any new treatments used by them are subjected to rigorous scientific testing including the 'double blind method' for example, the treatments given by Practitioners of Fringe Medicine are not subjected to such rigorous testing.

However, on the other hand Practitioners of the Complementary Medicines (as they prefer it to be called) reply that in the main their patients are those for whom orthodox medicine has failed and thus they are usually getting the 'difficult cases' with the simple ones having been cured by the doctors with orthodox medicine.

Against this, orthodox doctors are keen to point out that a considerable proportion of illnesses are psychological in origin and that any cure or alleviation has been brought about more by the confidence inspired by the Practitioner than on the methods employed. To which the Practitioners reply "Why then if the inspiration of confidence is all that is needed is this the monopoly of the Alternative Medical Practitioner?" And go on to ask why should the orthodox doctor, obviously no less capable of inspiring confidence attribute his cures to 'method' (not confidence) but attribute the cures of some of his failures to confidence (not method)?

Here then are the facts and opinions currently surrounding Complementary/Alterative/Fringe Medicine – call it what you will. For those with Tinnitus the position remains that orthodox medicine can but rarely offer any real alleviation, and certainly there is no known general cure.

Yet successful treatment of the associated symptoms such as depression, anxiety, irritation or suicidal tendencies certainly helps considerably to reduce the actual effect of the 'noises'.

It is a sad state of the art at the moment that certain of the various drugs offered by orthodox medicine in an effort to reduce the effect of these associated symptoms may often have certain side effects which cancel out any seemingly possible help the drug might be giving. No wonder the tinnitus sufferer should prefer to seek help from another source relatively free of such side effects. But here it must in all fairness be pointed out that some of the herbal remedies are very toxic, also some of the manipulations can sometimes do positive harm, as can acupuncture occasionally. Thus it would be wrong to endeavour to totally dissuade anyone from conventional drug treatment, for some depression when left untreated may well lead to suicide. This is surely all a matter of common sense on the part of the patients, to make their own decision.

ACUPUNCTURE

Numerous trials and attempts to treat Tinnitus by acupuncture have been made over the years, and a fair number of anecdotal and undocumented claims have been made regarding the success of this treatment. Unfortunately clinical evidence and closer scrutiny does not back up these claims.

If we are to assume, as do some, that Tinnitus is a 'pain in the auditory system' it is strange that although the clinical evidence shows it to be effective in painful conditions, serious trials on Tinnitus patients have shown a very poor record for Acupuncture. In fact it has been stated that professional acupuncture has no more effect than random needling so far as Tinnitus alleviation is concerned.

Some experts suggest that possibly trials embodying longer term active treatment might have shown some benefit, yet these do not appear to have been undertaken.

Marks *et al* in summing up a controlled trial of acupuncture in Tinnitus in which this relationship of Tinnitus to pain was examined, stated that statistical analysis of the group as a whole showed no apparent differences between placebo and active acupuncture treatment.

Over the past years I have been in contact with a considerable number of Tinnitus sufferers and know of many who, having been told by their doctors that there is no cure for the symptom immediately cast around seeking alleviation from one or other of the alternative medicines, one of the most popular being acupuncture. Yet I have still to meet a sufferer who has been cured of tinnitus by this treatment.

I am of course aware of the study carried out by Hanset *et al* in the comparison of true acupuncture and placebo acupuncture in a double-blind cross-over trial of Tinnitus patients who were otherwise resistant to treatment. These patients were reported to benefit equally in both groups, thus one can only conclude that the normal 'placebo effect' was operating rather than the treatment. It is unfortunate that the actual outcome of this study makes it practically impossible for any definite conclusions to be drawn one way or the other. However, one interesting point was made in the statement that some 30% of those who received real acupuncture spoke of 'some positive changes' during the study. But we must remember that 30% is the normal placebo effect.

The British Tinnitus Association report that there have been 'one' or 'two' cases of alleviation of tinnitus by acupuncture, but add the tinnitus in both these cases was of the intermittent type.

It would appear that the over-all impression given by those who have carried out careful experiments and tests in this particular field has been that acupuncture is capable of very little real effect so far as the alleviation of tinnitus is concerned.

ELECTRICAL STIMULATION

Efforts to alleviate Tinnitus by electrical stimulation were first attempted in the early 1800's following the invention of the first battery by Count Volta the Italian physicist from whom we have derived the, name 'volt' as a unit of electromotive force.

As has been previously mentioned Brenner (1868) tried to suppress Tinnitus by the use of electricity, and around 1890 MacNaughton-Jones used a small DC electrical current with one of the electrodes placed at the nape of the neck, and the other, a sponge-like electrode – placed in the ear. He was later to develop quite a complicated system of electrical stimulation for this purpose but it would appear that despite everything he found the results most disappointing.

There have been many other attempts since but nothing spectacular appears to have resulted. More recently House & Brackmann evaluated 29 cochlea-implant patients suffering from Tinnitus. House had noted that electrical stimulation in the cochlea produced suppression of Tinnitus in a few patients. He reported that electrical stimulation from the cochlea implant actually gave complete suppression in 8 of these patients (28%) and partial suppression in 15 patients (52%). And it is interesting to note that no patient's Tinnitus was at all exacerbated by this treatment.

It must be added however that electrical current can produce tissue damage. In one form the damage arises from ion deposits (electrically charged particles); these are more readily deposited by Direct Current (DC) than Alternating Current (AC). Fortunately AC can also have the effect of Tinnitus suppression. Using AC and a needle-type of electrode Graham & Hazell discovered that 2 of 9 patients so treated experienced short term relief from Tinnitus. For one of them the suppression lasted for four hours.

It is thought that C. J. C. Grapengiesser was probably the first to conduct any serious attempts to suppress tinnitus by electrical stimuli. This was in 1801, just a year after Volta invented the battery which stored DC current. The apparatus he used consisted of two electrodes composed of silver wire made into a small ball which was covered with a cloth moistened with water. It appears from the details of this experiment that it was able to suppress tinnitus and result in a residual inhibition lasting about four hours. However this method was soon dispensed with as it resulted in pain and nausea.

Later, three investigators, Hatton, Erulkar and Rosenberg tried filling the ear with saline into which one electrode was inserted, the other being placed on the mastoid on the same side. They tried several other spots for the second electrode but maintained the saline-filled ear in each experiment. They found that some 45% of their patients could receive tinnitus suppression by this method but it was not continued on the grounds that DC current is known to produce damage to the tissues, and an ear filled with saline hardly lends itself to any practical useage.

Other experiments followed with the placing of the electrode on the round window membrane and this effected suppression in 66% of cases. However, this effect ended with the switching off of the current. Also since only anodal (positive) current was effective it was concluded that the risk to tissue damage was too great to continue with this treatment.

Later, the development of Transcutaneous Electric Neural

Stimulation (TENS) for pain control produced some further experiments relating it to Tinnitus, and in the use of some TENS units there appeared to be no apparent tissue damage resulting.

These experiments, although effecting a certain relief with some patients, producing alleviation of even some hours duration following stimulation, unfortunately displayed rather a dismal success rate, and the final conclusion was that Transcutaneous Electrical Stimulation as carried out in these experiments was not an efficient therapy for Tinnitus.

A device known as a Theraband was brought out and commercially produced by the Audimaz Company which delivered a 60,000 Hz carrier wave modulated by a sweep frequency every 15 seconds. The latest reports seem to indicate that various and conflicting reports were obtained with this particular unit and that much more study is needed together with perhaps better standardisation of testing procedures.

A successful suppression of Tinnitus has been reported by Bauer using pulsed biphasic square wave D.C. giving successful suppression in 82% of the thirty patients tested. The stimulation lasted from 20 to 120 seconds only, with improvement enduring from 20 minutes up to even six months. But Vernon writes of this experiment 'Once again, these findings suggest that the variable results from one investigator to another may be due to patient population and/or selection, as well as stimulation procedures. Clearly, a great deal more work is needed in this area.'

Aran has also worked on electrical stimulation involving the round window membrane and the promontory, and Aran and Cazals using anodal DC (positive electrode) were able to obtain suppression in 60% of the patients undertaking the procedure when DC was applied to the round window membrane.

However, stimulation of the promontory obtained but partial suppression in only 43% of the patients. It was assumed that stimulation of the round window seems to provide a more direct path for the electrical current, their being able to report suppression in 87% of cases when applying anodal (positive) current to the round window.

There have also been studies of various 'wave forms' connected with electrical stimulation for Tinnitus suppression in America, but the conclusion has been that any additional work in this connection would have to be toward a more invasive procedure . . . the very thing that the experimentors had hoped to avoid.

Vernon and Fenwick summarise a report on "Attempts to Suppress Tinnitus with Transcutaneous Electrical Stimulation" as follows:

"Various electrical stimuli were tested for their ability to suppress Tinnitus Stimulation applied transdermally by electrodes placed on the preauricular and postauricular regions and on the two mastoids. Of the 50 patients tested, only 14 obtained relief that met the criterion of a reduction in the Tinnitus by 40% or more. When relief was obtained, it usually extended for several hours into the poststimulation period. There was only one positive response in the placebo trial, which was administered to all patients. It was concluded that transdermal electrical stimulation such as that used in this research is not a practical therapeutic procedure for the relief of Tinnitus".

AURICULOTHERAPY

I became very interested when a member of our Self Help Group announced that he was obtaining six and seven months Tinnitus alleviation from Auriculotherapy. He had been suffering badly from Meniere's Disease for some two years and his Tinnitus was of course consequent on this problem. The treatment he described, i.e. the holding of one electrode whilst the other was placed behind his ear, rather suggested Electrical Stimulation, but since he told me that the practitioner had spoken of special 'points' there appeared to have been an element of acupuncture involved.

Naturally, his report caused tremendous interest among the other Tinnitus sufferers in the Group, and two of them immediately volunteered to evaluate the treatment on behalf of the Group, as this is one of our aims.

One of these members took four sessions as prescribed from the same practitioner as the member reporting the treatment, with the use of electrodes as described. The other took four sessions with another practitioner who used acupuncture needles with electrical stimulation; the needles being placed not only in the region of the ear but in other parts of the body, thus producing a hybrid treatment between acupuncture and electrical stimulation. Unfortunately neither member was able to report the slightest improvement whatsoever in their tinnitus. This evaluation was in no way intended to be a clinically exhaustive test by any means, but merely a method of reporting on an experience which might well have been helpful to others.

There is in fact a British Institute of Auriculotherapy which issues a general information leaflet from which I quote, with their permission:

"According to traditional Chinese Medicine, the body meridians and vessels are our air and blood power structure – with the ear as the main central junction and crossroads of all these energy channels.

Auriculotherapy is based on the stimulation of individual acupuncture points in this area. Members of the Institute generally use Electronic Equipment to detect and stimulate these points. This method ensures accuracy, is extremely effective, and reassures those who fear pain or infection from the fine, sterile needles traditionally used.

Since 1951 French Physician Paul Nogier has conducted detailed studies on the correlation between the ear and other parts of the body, recognising in the structure of the ear a mirror image of its intro-uterine position – inverted, the head pointing downwards. Taking the inverted foetus as a guide to the first map of the ear and applying his research results to clinical treatment, Dr Nogier added new acupuncture points (there are now almost 200 known auricular points) and so became the foremost exponent and pioneer of auriculotherapy in the West.

Since its development by Nogier in the 1950's Auriculotherapy has increasingly been accepted by the medical profession worldwide. The ability to reduce dependence on drugs to control pain means that Patient exposure to side-effects is similarly reduced. This, together with the phenomenal success in the treatment of smoking and obesity in today's health-conscious society, more than justifies the recognition and increasing use of this Therapy.

The exceptional growth of Auriculotherapy in the United Kingdom prompted the formation of the British Institute of Auriculotherapy by a number of responsible practitioners. The BIA has since formulated a minimum requirement qualification in the form of written, oral and practical examinations.

Also required from any practicing Practitioner is the acceptance of, and adherence to a Code of Conduct. The most important part being that of referral with any medically questionable condition."

As will be seen, there is no specific reference to Tinnitus in this, although it certainly pays particular attention to the ear.

Chapter Six

Complementary Medicines in Tinnitus

PART TWO

COGNITIVE RESTRUCTURING

Macleod-Morgan, Court, and Roberts of the Flinders Psychology Clinic at Flinders University in South Australia carried out a most interesting 'treatment' for tinnitus sufferers in the early part of the 1980s, involving Cognitive Restructuring.

This is a mixture of relaxation and imagery aimed at teaching an altered perception of chronic tinnitus to a number of patients. All these patients had previously received medical attention that had been entirely ineffective.

Following a number of visits to the Clinic those very noises which had so been troubling them, and so interfering with the quality of their lives, became a cue for peace and relaxation. Thus did the tinnitus become something to be welcomed whereas prior to this it had been feared.

The reports of this particular attempt for the alleviation of tinnitus certainly makes interesting reading.

One woman of forty-three was referred with serious tinnitus problems, together with vertigo and bad depression. She had undergone various investigations by Ear Nose & Throat Specialists, had auditory tests in which it was found her hearing was normal, and had received drug treatment all to no avail.

She also reported reluctant sessions of hypnotherapy. With slight hypnotic induction she was introduced to relaxation with the suggestion of a pleasant scene on a sunny beach. She aroused herself from this and was then reassured that the therapy would only proceed in short steps entirely at the pace which she set herself.

On her second visit she agreed on the exploration of a light trance and cognitive and other interventions aimed at her depression were introduced, and these continued with her subsequent visits together with hypnotic intervention. Throughout all visits emphasis was placed on the fact that she was able to arouse herself at any time and was asked to raise her right finger as a signal if at any time she felt uneasy.

On her third visit she stated that she was feeling the most depressed when her vertigo was at its worst. On this, hypnosis was induced with the suggestion that there was a safe place for her to go to where she would be totally in control. Following this the idea of a dashboard with two control knobs was introduced, one was for the control of her Tinnitus, and the other for the control of her balance.

She was obviously obtaining an excellent visualization of the dashboard and she described in some detail what it was like. She was then told to turn up the Tinnitus knob to what (to her) seemed to be a maximum level, and then down again, She described the 'control knobs'. The Tinnitus one was set at zero and the vertigo one precisely mid-way which indicated perfect balance. After suggestion for successful practice at home, she aroused herself.

At her following visit she reported a certain amount of success, but appeared to be worried concerning the 'balance knob' feeling that this might come off its mid-way calibration, and she not be able to shift it. Here help was given her by the suggestion that she moved the knob forward and thus felt in control of it. But at this stage she complained of head pain and pain in the ear, and so the suggestion was made for her to return to the 'safe place' and then arouse herself.

At later visits she again spoke of her fear of losing control of the balance knob, but this was finally resolved by the suggestion that she visualized the knob as clicking into place and that it could only be moved by pulling it out and turning it. With further reinforcement of her successful control, it was possible to end the therapy after only nine visits.

Of this particular example of case history it was said that as regards the tinnitus this woman was sensitized to, it was due to psychological difficulties. It would appear that previous attempts to help her had failed to take these other difficulties into consideration.

A further case, that of a woman of 60 is also contained in this report. She had been referred by her GP and had suffered from tinnitus for ten years. She had been seen by four ear specialists and had been supplied with a hearing aid. She had suffered depressive breakdowns and had been given ECT which had resulted in some memory loss. She was a well educated woman who had previously worked as a secretary.

Her first few visits were extremely difficult as she seemed quite unable to attempt any form of relaxation. However, after a while, almost from her own suggestion she was able to visualize a peaceful rose garden to which she even made further suggestions of a hammock to lie in and the sweet scent of 'Peace' roses.

For various reasons the 'control knob' suggestion was dropped with this patient and the rose garden idea developed. After a while she was able to obtain a deep state of relaxation whilst listening to the voice of a popular tenor following the suggestion that her tinnitus was really the basis of some lovely music.

From here on she quickly progressed and discontinued therapy after nine visits on the suggestion of the therapists. She left delighted with her success and skill in relaxation and her control over her tinnitus which had given her new-found confidence.

COGNITIVE THERAPY

The idea of Cognitive Therapy was originally born in the United States arising from the works of Albert Ellis and Aaron Beck. It endeavours to identify certain attitudes and irrational beliefs which so often stand in the way of the solving of problems. So very often a person's Tinnitus is exacerbated by their attitude towards it. So often emotional reactions are the root cause of many of the associated symptoms.

The therapy has already been used most successfully in the treatment of various emotional disorders. In the application to Tinnitus it has proved successful in enabling people to alter their attitude towards 'the noises' and to regard their Tinnitus in a different light. In thus changing irrational beliefs, the accompanying depression, anxiety and general emotional distress is reduced considerably with the result that eventually a person is able to cope with the problem which actually becomes less noticeable.

In this connection I quote by permission from the report of Dr Ross Coles on a weekend course run by Dr Richard Hallam and Mr Simon Jakes in March 1987 at Debden House, Loughton, Essex, and which appeared in The Sound Barrier of December 1987.

"It started on the Friday evening with a description of each of the five participants attending, of his own Tinnitus and its effects on his life. Next morning the tutors explained the relationship between Tinnitus and its effects, the latter often being worsened or even created by the sufferer's beliefs about the cause, nature, and future effects of Tinnitus rather than by the Tinnitus itself.

Cognitive Therapy is directed toward greater understanding (cognition) of how these beliefs cause much of the distress that Tinnitus sufferers experience, and how this suffering may be reduced by appropriate challenge of these beliefs and replacement of them by more realistic and less fearful attitudes.The treatment aims to alter a person's subjective experience of their tinnitus.

Then came the essential A – B – C concept of cognitive therapy. Sufferers can easily describe C – the consequences of their Tinnitus such as tension, fear, depression, and they can often identify A the Activating event or events which may lead to these Consequences. Less easy to realise, sometimes needing skilful probing by the therapist is B – the Beliefs that link the Activating Event to the Consequences, but these are usually revealed by asking why the sufferer thinks a particular Activating Event appeared to cause the consequences described. These Beliefs and Consequences were discussed to consider to what extent they may be true, sensible or likely.

At this stage the idea of reverse role-playing was introduced by the tutors, using themselves as examples at first. The idea is to challenge your own beliefs when they are acted out by someone else. It works like this. Smith describes his Tinnitus to Jones in terms of its Activating events and Consequences. Smith then starts to question Jones [acting as Smith] as to the Beliefs which link the Activating events and Consequences. He then goes on to challenge these Beliefs with questions intended to see if the Beliefs are as certainly true as they may seem to be or whether they are not tinged with (unjustified) pessimism. He also questions the feared Consequences, – are they really likely – are they so awful – could he really not manage, and so on?

The Report continues: 'It took all of us ... quite a time to grasp what was happening in the role-playing. At first it was mildly annoying as it seemed an unnecessary and unreal thing to do. But then the penny dropped – admittedly with some help from the tutors, by way of explanation.

Role-playing is helpful, even essential, because if any of us had challenged Smith directly he would have immediately been put on the defensive, thus tending to reinforce his beliefs rather than to modify them. But by having Smith challenge Jones (acting as Smith) it meant that Smith was in effect not only challenging his own beliefs but doing so in a very constructive way. The partners in the role-play took it in turns to have their beliefs challenged in this way.

This role-playing activity continued with participants working in pairs, supervised and assisted by the tutors. But before the course was over, we had a session of relaxation therapy to teach the participants how to relax in the presence of stress. This was then coupled with a trial of imagery and distraction techniques designed to get the person to think of the cause (tinnitus) of his stress experience in a different and more pleasant light; to help him concentrate on other sounds, such as the ticking of a clock, so as to reduce his attention on his Tinnitus, and finally to imagine the Tinnitus or the external sound gradually becoming less loud.

On departure I think that all the participants felt better about their Tinnitus, understanding better its nature, its effects and how to control or reduce these effects by change of attitude. The only pity was that the course was not longer, or could not be followed up locally.

As will be seen, Cognitive Restructuring has as its basis, a patient's own personal imagery and is able to alleviate tinnitus by pushing it to the end of the 'perceptual queue'. However, this technique demands considerable effort from the patient as well as a willingness and the ability to suspend disbelief.

One great advantage of this particular technique is that the patient is trained in self control which can so easily become enhanced with practice.

It is suggested that possible imageries that might be suggested could include running water, splashing fountains, and music.

The report ends by pointing out that by teaching patients to make peace and not war with tinnitus, and by drawing on their own resources of creativity and motivation, much of their discomfort can be alleviated.

YOGA

Yoga is a complete way of life evolved in India over thousands of years. Up to twenty or so years ago, anyone practicing it would have been looked upon as somewhat eccentric but in the West today it is widely practiced and accepted.

Individual tuition and Yoga classes can be found in practically every town these days and although up to a few years ago mostly women took it up, today more and more men are enjoying it and finding it a great help in the management of stress.

Since anxiety, stress, depression and general debilitation can so often plague the Tinnitus sufferer as associated symptoms, Yoga is now being recommended by most specialists in the management of Tinnitus. It can be practiced by people of all ages and stages of life. It can help in the prevention, cure and management of a wide range of disorders both physical and psychological and should be seriously considered by anyone who finds their Tinnitus spoiling the quality of their life.

The deep relaxation obtainable by Yoga is one of its finest benefits for Tinnitus sufferers. The fundamental techniques are best learned from a qualified Yoga teacher, although there is no shortage of books, videos and cassettes on the subject from which one can learn a lot oneself. It is essential that Yoga be practiced regularly at least for half an hour a day; for certain difficult conditions over an hour a day. However, the time spent in its practice is said to be well balanced by the fact that it reduces one's sleeping time.

HOMEOPATHY

With such scant help available from orthodox medical sources it is hardly surprising that so many people suffering from Tinnitus turn to other possible sources of help. Yet it is possible that your own GP in these days may well have had some training in

---

Note: Homoeopathy or Homeopathy – either spelling is accepted.

Homeopathy, and since homeopathic medicines are available on the Health Service and there are specific treatments within Homeopathy for various types of Tinnitus it is felt that readers would be interested in more information on this particular fringe medicine.

The basic principle behind homeopathy is 'Let like be treated by like'. It was a theory put forward by Hippocrates (400 BC) who quoted several examples. The same theories were put forward by Paracelsus in the Middle Ages.

Indeed it was Hippocrates who pointed to the healing power of Nature and the duty of every physician to be Nature's intermediary. Unfortunately this philosophy was completely reversed by Galen (AD 131–201) whose aims were to destroy the disease and thus subdue Nature. These ideas then became systemized as allopathy with all its confused ideas and horrendous methods such as purgation, bleeding, and use of drugs many of which were potentially poisonous. This was summed up well by Boerhave (1668–1738) when he remarked 'It would have been better for mankind had physicians never existed!'

Some twenty years after Boerhave's death Samuel Hahnemann was born, who graduated as Doctor of Medicine in 1799. Totally dissatisfied with the medical methods of his day he gave up his practice and concentrated solely on his own system of medicine which he called Homeopathy.

In complete contrast to the medical practices of his day, Hahnemann would administer only one single drug the action of which was well known. No repeat doses were to be given unless the symptoms of the illness reappeared. At all times the very smallest possible dosage was administered in order to minimise any reactions.

In Homeopathy the potency principle is always intriguing. For example if a poison such as bella-donna is to be used medically it is essential that the dose be very small indeed. On the principles of Hahnemann one grain of the substance is to be mixed with nine parts of alcohol and shaken vigorously. Then one part of this first dilution similarly diluted and shaken results in a 2× potency; serial dilutions to any number may be made. In this manner 1 in 100 dilutions are known as 2c (2cH) and 1 in 1000 dilutions 1M. The most usual potencies include 3× 5× 6c 30c 200c 1M and 10M.

Homeopathic treatment is perfectly safe and although there may be a slight aggravation of symptoms following a remedy this is usually of very short duration and is in fact a sign that this particular remedy should be effective.

Being an holistic medicine a visit to a Homeopathic Doctor can sometimes be a somewhat lengthy affair since it is necessary for the practitioner to obtain a comprehensive picture of both you and your symptoms including details of your mental and emotional state (all too often ignored in allopathy) but vital for successful homeopathic prescription.

SUGGESTED HOMOEOPATHIC REMEDIES FOR VARIOUS TYPES OF TINNITUS

Noises louder on waking	Lachesis
Humming noise & headache	Kali Phos.
Tinnitus & Recruitment	Actaea Rac
Tinnitus with vertigo & sickness	Carbo Vegetabilis
Tinnitus with catarrh	Pulsatilla
Difficulty getting to sleep	Aconite
Tinnitus worse at night	Graphites
Buzzing type of Tinnitus	China Officinalis
Buzzing Tinnitus with slight vertigo	Chininum Sulphuricum
Crackling noises in the ears	Kali Carbonium
Fluttering noises in the ears	Platinum
Hissing types of Tinnitus	Digitalis
Humming sounds (without headache)	Lycopodium
High ringing sound	Causticum
Roaring noises in the head & ears	Baryta Carbonica
A rushing sound resembling wind	Kali Carbonium
A sound like the sea	Chamomilla Vularis
A squashing noise on swallowing	Calcarea Carbonica
Depression (for men)	Ignatia
Depression (for women)	Sepia
Irritability	Bryonia
Migraine (associated with Tinnitus)	Kalium Bichromicum
Lack of Concentration	Apis mel

Since Homoeopathic Medicines are easy to administer and completely safe for all, including infants, the pregnant and the elderly and are in addition very easily obtainable from one's chemist, readers with Tinnitus may welcome some suggestions for a First Aid Trial! These suggestions have been given me by a prominent Homoeopathic Doctor.

All should be in 6c potency and two tablets taken three times a day. These should be taken with a clean tongue and with the mouth free from the effects of peppermint, toothpaste or tobacco and well before or after food and drink. No coffee should be taken during the treatment as this is thought to negate the action of the remedy. Place the tablets under the tongue and allow them to dissolve naturally.

Most Pharmacists dealing in Homeopathic Remedies will be only too pleased to advise you on any problems.

BIOFEEDBACK

The origin of the technique of Biofeedback dates back to W. G. Walter's research in the 1950's on the electrical rhythms of the brain. Whilst observing a patient listening to a football match on the radio he noticed that the alpha rhythms of the brain appeared to respond directly with the fortunes of his favourite football team. However it was J. Kamiya of the USA who later discovered in 1958 that it was possible for patients to consciously control their own alpha rhythms when given certain information.

Research continued and it was discovered that certain animals could be taught to make one ear warmer and the other cooler by the use of biofeedback and that humans could learn to voluntarily control their muscle tension, heart rate, and other responses. Very soon small hand-temperature meters, electrical skin resistance meters etc were appearing on the market.

Briefly, the procedures used in Biofeedback techniques are designed to give a patient control over a psychological variable of which they have not been aware of having such control.

It should be understood from the outset that no amount of Biofeedback will have the effect of teaching a person how to reduce their actual Tinnitus but will certainly teach them how to relax properly. Thus it is an effective addition to therapy, although not a therapy in its own right. It is compatible with all the usual relaxation techniques as it is with most forms of counselling.

The use of Biofeedback equipment together with a physical technique [for example, breath control], or a psychological one [such as analysis], helps a patient to learn to discover the true causes of their response to stress. However, few Practitioners of biofeedback would suggest that Tinnitus is affected in any way with biofeedback sessions but that it enables a patient to gain control over general relaxation and thus results in making the tinnitus more tolerable.

It would be of great benefit to Tinnitus sufferers if some form of Biofeedback with an objective acoustical basis could be found which would enable the patient to control the magnitude of the Tinnitus in the same way as blood pressure and muscle tension are possible. To date I know of no such technique.

Training in Biofeedback is given singly or in groups. The interaction experienced in group training does appear to be an aid in learning.

Certainly Biofeedback training does appear to offer some hope to Tinnitus sufferers, although it does seem that any resulting improvements so far as Tinnitus is concerned is probably more due to an increase in the ability to cope with the symptom than to any true reduction in the noises.

Let us hope that in the future more tinnitus-related methods of Biofeedback training may be discovered and developed.

HYPNOTHERAPY

Although I have been personally aware of a number of Tinnitus sufferers obtaining considerable help from hypnosis, such help has essentially been connected with the associated symptoms such as depression, anxiety, stress, and irritability etc and has to my knowledge had no actual effect on the Tinnitus itself. The usual treatments have consisted of a session with the Hypnotherapist followed by the daily use of a short audio-tape giving details of self-hypnosis embodying complete muscular and mental relaxation.

It should be emphasised that there is nothing sinister in

hypnosis – no one can be hypnotised if they do not wish to be, and self-hypnosis is not a difficult discipline to acquire.

Normally, the first time a person is hypnotised or uses self-hypnosis only a shallow trance is achieved but with practice one can deepen these states of trance at will.

Certainly there is a place for hypnosis in Tinnitus management as it applies to stress and other aspects but there is no evidence that it can have much effect on the Tinnitus itself.

CHIROPRACTIC

Chiropractic treats mechanical disorders of the joints, especially the spinal joints. Many of these mechanical disorders are closely related to our style of living today. They result above all from sitting for long periods at desks or in cars, on unsuitable seating, and also from incorrect bending and lifting habits.

Treatment is gentle and painless and very much safer than taking drugs for the pain or trying to carry on as normal and ignoring Nature's warnings. Latest estimates give the number of skilled practitioners currently at work worldwide as forty thousand.

All qualified Chiropractors undergo intensive training and very many of them work within state health care systems.

The origins of chiropractic are closely allied to osteopathy, both being manipulative practices and involving an element of preventive care.

However, a Chiropractor tends to use less leverage and will manipulate directly over a joint in a precise direction; an Osteopath will generally use more leverage but makes the adjustment further away from the joint being treated.

Chiropractic first came to the fore in 1895 independent of general medicine. It was developed by David Palmer (1845–1913) who discovered the power of spinal manipulation. By adjustment of the vertebrae in the neck area he treated a patient for chronic deafness.

He was convinced that the basis of disease was in the spine, and developed the theory that displaced ('subluxed') vertebrae restricted the spinal nerves, interfering with the flow of nervous energy through the body. At one time his theories were rejected by orthodox medicine despite the fact that his views were in line with medical research of that time. Today, Palmer's original ideas are not regarded as gospel although Chiropractors are still primarily spinal experts.

As an independent branch of medicine Chiropractic has often been challenged to prove its worth. It has for a long time maintained that its theories regarding skeletal function were correct. These theories were until quite recently hotly disputed by orthodox medicine. For instance Chiropractic contends that bad movement and weight-bearing speed up degeneration of the framework of the body, and that spinal discs can be treated by manipulation. These beliefs have since been supported by both detailed medical research, and clinical trials, and studies confirm the effectiveness of this therapy.

As regards the application of Chiropractic in Tinnitus alleviation, I have before me the case history of a young woman who was suddenly hit by horrendous noises in the head and ears. 'It's like a road drill' she shouted, pacing up and down and banging the right side of her head with her hand. After visiting her GP and two eminent ear specialists followed by various other tests and efforts to help her, some eighteen months later the noises were still there and she was becoming very debilitated.

It was at this point that a television programme introduced her to Chiropractic and she decided to consult a Chiropractor. He took a very full case history and made a thorough examination of her neck. He discovered that her neck was slightly distorted and assured her that this distortion was not only causing the Tinnitus but also the pains, pins and needles, and sometimes the feeling of complete deadness in the side of her face and head.

X-rays were taken of her neck and back which immediately disclosed a definite curve in the neck and several abnormalities in the vertebrae.

It was explained to her that the head (often weighing some 25 lbs) had to be supported by the muscles and neck joints, and these must work perfectly in order to do so; when they did not, then the symptoms she had described usually presented themselves.

Following one short session of manipulation and massage her Tinnitus became much quieter, whilst the pains and discomfort in her head were less frequent. Within three visits, spread over eight weeks from the original appointment, she was cured.

It must however be added that the Tinnitus DID return some eight months later. She consulted the Chiropractor again and reported having a filling in a tooth the day previous to the Tinnitus coming on again. She states that he took her jaw firmly in his hands and twisted it just a little to the left. And since that day she has had permanent peace in her head.

Chapter Seven
Tinnitus Maskers

From way back in the thirteenth century a quotation comes to us asking why it is that if one has a 'buzzing in the ears' a further sound stops it? Is it that greater sound can drive away the lesser? There is nothing new in this idea, and man has experimented on these lines at various times ever since in his efforts to alleviate Tinnitus but with little real success. It would appear that there is an interesting analogy here with Homoeopathy in 'like curing like'.

Jones & Knudsen in 1928 brought out what was possibly the first electrical Tinnitus Masker but this was only a fairly crude type of harmonic generator and not very successful. However great strides have been made in this field of late and the modern Tinnitus Masker now resembles a small hearing aid which is placed either in or behind the ear. The simpler type which fit behind the ear comprise a tiny generator producing 'white noise' combined with various filters and an amplifier and transducer.

There are also Maskers which are programmable but these require a larger (body-worn) device. Additionally a type of Masker known as a Tinnitus Instrument combining both Masker and Hearing Aid is available. Unfortunately not every Tinnitus sufferer is able to benefit from the use of a masker, and of course it would be useless to attempt to use one if you had no hearing whatever in the offending ear.

Between 1977 and 1979 Hazell & Wood reported that of the first 148 Maskers fitted between those dates there was a failure rate of no less than 60% and only 12% reported any continuous relief at all. This suggested to them that obviously considerable counselling and follow-up visits to the hospital were vitally necessary. And indeed by this means the next 142 patients fitted with maskers resulted in an acceptance rate of no less than 81%! It was however stated that the degree of relief obtained from

Tinnitus by the masking varied considerably between patients and also from time to time in the same patients.

There has certainly been one 'spin off' from the introduction of Maskers and that is an effect known as 'residual inhibition' i.e. periods of varying length in which a patient obtains total Tinnitus relief on removing the Masker after use.

If a Consultant suggests that a Masker might suit you it is certainly wise to give it a trial, but one can only judge these things from personal contact and experience, and in my own case I fear I found a Masker quite useless, and in my contacts with many dozens of Tinnitus sufferers I have the feeling that despite the fact that many Maskers have been fitted, there are a great number of these to be found unused in drawers!

Total 'residual inhibition' HAS been achieved in a small percentage of cases but neither Hazell nor Vernon now recommend that patients should be counselled on the likelihood of this happening.

Why substituting yet another noise for the Tinnitus noise should serve as an effective relief for some patients has been explained in several different ways. Some sufferers tell us that their 'tonal' or 'narrowband' Tinnitus is far more annoying than the 'broadband' sound from the masker. Another feature which has been mentioned by some patients is the fact that the masker is a 'real sound' which is under their control, whilst the Tinnitus sound is not.

This is rather in line with the fact that quite a number of patients experience relief from Tinnitus when fitted with a satisfactory hearing aid, for in such cases the environmental noises are amplified and thus drown out the Tinnitus noise.

Before a Masker can be fitted a personal ear mould has to be made taken from a mould impression. The majority of patients prefer a mould of the 'open' type which does not occlude the ear canal. A solid or badly vented mould is inclined to give the impression of an ear plug even before the masker is switched on which gives the impression of the Tinnitus sounding louder. This has been one of the most common causes of Masker failure.

The open mould is additionally useful by reason of the fact that it helps the high frequency and does not interfere so much with the hearing in quiet surroundings. However with considerable hearing loss or very severe Tinnitus a mould that occludes the ear may be necessary but even then a vent adjacent to the ear canal is best provided.

Possibly originating from anger against the continuous noise of the Tinnitus (for irritability is one of the commonly associated symptoms) some patients are inclined to increase the volume of their Masker, feeling that it might result in extirpating some physical defect in their hearing mechanism which is to their mind causing the Tinnitus. But since so much Tinnitus is originally noise-induced in the first place, this is extremely unwise.

Unfortunately, for varying reasons certain cases of Tinnitus cannot be masked. Take for example a person whose hearing loss is so great that the sound of the masker even at top intensity gives insufficient sensation to the frequency region or site of the Tinnitus. Similar unmaskability can occur in cases where although there is sufficient hearing a masker does not work no matter what the intensity. The reasons for this do not appear at present to be fully understood. In such a case as the latter very often the use of a Walkman stereo with suitable music will be found helpful. Further details of this will be found in Chapter Eight.

RESIDUAL INHIBITION (RI)

This is a phenomenon that was first reported by Spalding in 1903 although not known by the name Residual Inhibition until around 1977. Often following the termination of effective masking a patient's Tinnitus was found to not immediately reappear at the same intensity as it was before masking. Indeed, with some patients it would disappear completely for varying periods of time, usually of short duration.

Early reports of RI raised great hopes in the American Tinnitus circles as the reports of patients claiming extended durations of the phenomenon reached the press. Indeed, numerous unproven expectations were created by various garbled versions of its

---

At the time of going to press clinical trials funded by the Hearing Research Trust at Manchester University's Audiological Technology Unit are enabling researchers to assess the benefits of a remarkable new earmould material called Otana.

A soft acrylic-based resin, Otana enables earmoulds to be produced in a single stage process without the need for sophisticated tools. It is explained that at the moment customised earmoulds are produced using a two-stage process but it is very difficult to make an earmould fit accurately using this technique.

effects. In reporting various periods of alleviation or relief, hours – days – and even instances of complete cures appeared in the national press. All this had the effect of creating totally unrealistic expectations among both patients and practitioners.

Today, although there has been considerable study undertaken on the subject of RI it is still confusing the experts. Certainly it is there, but they are unable to discover the factors which influence it.

Vernon categorically states that 88% of patients attending the Oregon Clinic experience RI. Although there are cases of patients obtaining fairly long periods of relief following masking, and even a few reported 'cures' these instances are very rare indeed. However one helpful 'spin-off' from this discovery has been that those patients who show Residual Inhibition have been found to be far more likely to profit from Masking than those who do not. Additionally there is every indication that the type of Tinnitus which results from such things as industrial noise exposure seems to give better results of RI than other forms.

It is a strange fact that in the case of those patients obtaining complete Residual Inhibition the Tinnitus does not reappear gradually but 'bounces back in intermittent spurts' which is contrary to what one would anticipate.

A further interesting fact is that RI is not obtainable through the use of hearing aids, despite the fact that in certain cases hearing aids can be used to mask out the Tinnitus. The phenomenon only occurs following the use of a masker. It is thus felt that environmental sounds are possibly not sufficiently continuous.

In 1984 Harris & Mollestrom discovered that the best method of producing Residual Inhibition was to closely imitate the actual sounds of the Tinnitus itself so far as was possible, and to this end they produced a programmable type of masker.

Hazell sums up the whole matter of RI in pointing out that with masking technique as it stands at present, particularly with narrow or broad-band noise, it would be very unfair to allow a patient to be too hopeful of achieving the phenomenon. He does suggest that some 10% could achieve short periods of freedom, and between 30% & 40% periods of reduced intensity of their Tinnitus, following masking.

Since Residual Inhibition at least achieves SOME relief, and so far as is known is free of any side effects whatever, it is surely worthy of considerable further research, test and study? If it could be used to effect reasonably long periods of relief (say weeks or months) this would be the answer to the dream of every Tinnitus sufferer.

Chapter Eight

The Power of Music

Music as we know it today is only around 800 years old, yet its actual origins lie deep in the mists of time. Primitive man firmly believed that musical sound was the work of some supernatural being, and various forms of music were used in all the ancient rites. Unfortunately, as with so many other things in life, although its powers can be used to very good effect, these same powers can so easily be abused. In fact it is very doubtful if its full importance on both counts are generally realised.

One of the present approaches in the many attempts at tinnitus alleviation is by filtered music on tape through a personal stereo such as a Walkman. This has been of particular interest to me. For some 50 or so years I have been in close contact with music and musicians and have had the privilege of knowing many of the finest musicians in the world, especially on the stringed instrument side.

Since becoming personally involved with hearing loss and tinnitus, I have, in looking back realised what a great number of these performers, so actively and prominently engaged in the making of organised sound throughout their careers eventually seemed to develop various hearing difficulties. This has led me to wonder whether there might not be some connection between the active performance of music and these auditory difficulties. For my own part, I vividly recall that the first warning I had of anything being amiss with my own hearing was whilst playing the violin in a Symphony Orchestra during which I found every beat from the timpani becoming absolute agony [recruitment].

Surely there can be no greater tragedy for a musician than hearing loss, for hearing is the very sense that binds musicians to their art?

When one looks back into musical history, it is amazing to discover so many reports of deafness and tinnitus among even the musical giants of the past. I have sometimes wondered whether perhaps the hearing mechanism of a musician is by nature more finely attuned and thus more liable to degeneration or damage than that of others, possibly exacerbated by the intense listening, study and practice of the art.

It is not difficult to recall quite a number of great musicians who were beset by deafness and tinnitus, and there is one particular example in which one of them introduced the sound of his tinnitus into one of his compositions.

This written in 1876 acts as a memorial from a tinnitus sufferer of all those years ago, telling us not only that this disability is nothing new, but that even in spite of it one is able to reach the pinnacle of one's aspirations with sufficient determination.

I suppose the finest example of these famous musicians suffering from these auditory difficulties would be Ludwig von Beethoven (1770–1827) who in a letter to his old friend Dr Wegeler gives us a clear report of obvious tinnitus when he wrote 'My ears buzz and hum day and night – I can tell you that I lead a most miserable life!' He then proceeds to give us a classic example of recruitment when he says 'I can hear sounds it is true, but cannot make out the words, and if anyone shouts I just cannot bear it!'

At times he used an old fashioned ear trumpet. It was an ornamental brass affair with a small curved pipe at the hearing end and a bell-like trumpet at the other end. It is today on display in a museum in Vienna. At one stage he reported having 'treatment' for his ears at one of the then finest hospitals in Vienna. This comprised almond oil being poured in his ears and being ordered to take several ice cold baths a day together with some other equally absurd recommendations. Needless to report, none of this was of any use at all.

Franz Schubert (1797–1828) like his contemporary Beethoven also suffered with deafness and from the few meagre reports we have we can conclude that he also had tinnitus which has been associated with his isolated lifestyle. His problems, with all the depressive and debilitating effects are well exemplified in his Fifth Symphony (The Tragic) the slow movement of which is particularly tinged with melancholy.

Robert Schumann (1810–1856) soon after his 40th birthday spoke of 'remarkable aural symptoms' followed by the persistent sounding of the note 'A' in both his ears, and thus quite definitely had tinnitus. Some two years later he wrote of 'very strong and painful aural afflictions' which grew steadily worse, and he had the illusion of hearing music constantly in his head. About a week later he become suicidal with it and suddenly ran out of his lodging house to the Rhine Bridge and threw himself into the river. Some fishermen eventually saved his life and took him home, and this is possibly one of the earliest recorded instances of someone attempting suicide because of tinnitus.

Vaughan Williams (1872–1958) first became aware of his hearing difficulties rather late in life, and somehow managed to conduct by using a hearing aid, but in private he preferred a form of ear trumpet (which he named his 'coffee pot') and which he found gave a more realistic musical sound than did the electrical aid of his day.

Robert Franz (1815–1892) was a famous German Organist, Conductor, and Composer who wrote "I most suddenly became completely deaf and most troubled by a horrendous noise in my ears and extreme irritability to any loud sounds".

Gabriel Faure (1854–1924) became extremely deaf at middle age and also suffered badly from tinnitus coupled with pitch distortion resulting in the higher notes in music sounding flat and low notes sharp. It is a phenomenon reported by numbers of musicians in these days of electronic music.

Smetana (1824–1884) was another composer referred to earlier as the one who introduced the actual sound of his tinnitus into one of his compositions – the Finale of his String Quartet in E minor (No 1) which is entitled 'From my life'. An entry in his diary dated July 28th 1874 reads 'My hearing is failing and at the same time my head seems to be spinning and I feel giddy'. He continues to write of his first string quartet and explains 'In this I had to give a tone picture of my life. In the first movement my leaning toward art in my youth, the romantic atmosphere, the inexpressible longing for something I could neither express nor define, and also the presage as it were of my future misfortune and the long insistent note, the one in the Finale grew out of this beginning. It is that fateful ringing of high-pitched tones in my ear which in 1874 announced the beginning of my deafness. I allowed myself this little play because for me it was so prophetic'.

Later he was to write 'Deafness would be a relatively decent condition if only all was quiet in my head. But the greatest torture is caused me by the almost continuous internal noise which goes on in my head and sometimes rises to thunderous crashing'.

The examples quoted represent but a small proportion of the actual vast number of musicians who have reported such difficulties in the past but the advent of electronic music has caused almost an epidemic in these problems.

For those readers who would like further information on the therapeutic value of music related to Tinnitus I would recommend the book by Patricia Joudry *Sound Therapy for the Walkman* published in Canada and with a foreword by Yehudi Menuhin the famous violinist. This covers the new discovery concerning the effect of sound upon the brain. The technique involves listening to specially prepared tapes on a personal stereo such as a WALKMAN. The tapes are easy listening, and need no concentration. Additionally, the beneficial effects are said to be absorbed at very low volume and the personal stereo can be worn during all usual activities if required.

One of the documented results is the alleviation of disorders which stem from the imbalance of inner ear fluid, nausea, dizziness and tinnitus.

This therapy is known as Audio-Psycho-Phonology and is based on the work of Dr A. A. Tomatis, a prominent French ENT Specialist.

Other forms of medicinal music are now common in the treatments used in many neurological departments, and indeed are looked upon as a major form of treatment to which patients with problems of behaviour, neurosis, and even mental deficiency have been found to respond most favourably.

Now that the use of Medicinal Music has reached those of us suffering from auditory difficulties, let us hope that it may eventually prove successful in this particular field as well.

Chapter Nine

Depression

We are all subject to minor swings in mood, but when a depressed mood becomes persistent and begins to interfere with a person's daily life, then a depressive illness is developing.

Perhaps it would be helpful here to discuss some of the ways in which Depression may be detected in its early stages. Its arrival is usually so insidious that it is rarely recognised by the victim. In pointing out some of the warning signs it may help to alert a spouse or friend to precisely what is happening, and by persuading the person concerned to seek help, save much unhappiness later on.

Since here we are essentially concerned with Depression as related to Tinnitus, let us first try to discover precisely WHY this is so prevalent among people with Tinnitus.

We experience three differing levels of hearing. Primitive, Warning and Symbolic. Primitive Hearing refers to the normal environmental sounds about us. Much of this is experienced subconsciously. Warning Hearing refers to any signal in sound such as someone calling 'Look out!' or the sound of an approaching vehicle. In other words any sound which we instinctively recognise as being one of impending danger. Finally, Symbolic Hearing refers to our use of sound in communication as for example in conversation.

It is when we experience interference with out Primitive Hearing such as occurs with the reduction or complete loss of our hearing, or the heavy interference brought on by severe Tinnitus, that we can so easily develop Depression. These sounds form the whole background of life as we know it, enabling us to experience participation in our environment and indeed in our whole world as we know it.

With this ability absent or even badly restricted, as happens with severe Tinnitus or hearing loss, the situation develops into a profound feeling of isolation. Add to this the additional weight of loneliness – as in the case of those living alone, and we have the typical picture of so many people's lives in which the sufferer feels totally out of touch, unwanted, unloved, and deeply depressed in consequence.

Should you suspect that someone with whom you live is suffering from depression, what are the early warning signs? Probably the most significant is that the person loses interest and enjoyment in almost every aspect of life. Such a change as this is very quickly noticed by other people – especially those close to them.

I will give just some of the symptoms that may be apparent. It must not be assumed every sufferer from depression will experience ALL these symptoms at the same time. The coverage given is a general one.

Firstly a depressed person finds everything an effort. Usually they just cannot be bothered. There is usually a change in appetite pattern. Some have but little inclination to eat; others are inclined to over-eat. They may tell you that they 'cannot think straight' and cannot concentrate. Their memory is often affected.

There is usually a change in attitude to their work, whether this be at home or out at work. There is a lack of interest in sports and hobbies that they have previously always enjoyed. There is a loss of libido or sexual appetite which can of course so easily lead to marital problems, creating still further difficulties for them. Often there will be fits of crying although they will be unable to tell you the reason.

Their general lack of interest may well extend to personal hygiene and their general personal appearance. Some completely neglect themselves in these respects. Sleep patterns also are usually affected. There will be both difficulty in actually getting off to sleep, and of waking early in the mornings – say around 3 to 4 am and being unable to get off to sleep again.

There are usually complaints of various physical symptoms such as headaches, back aches, stomach troubles, tight feelings in the chest, giddiness and blurred vision.

Most people when depressed are additionally apathetic and often unwilling to seek professional help. It is therefore up to others to try to persuade them to seek such help (unpopular as the suggestion may prove!).

There are two kinds of depressive illness. One is known as Endogenous Depression – a type which is formed from within and comes from no external cause. The other kind is known as Reactive Depression which results from the reaction of a person to difficult circumstances, and this includes mourning.

The incidence of depression may well be judged by a recent study of 2,225 consecutive patients attending a North London Health Centre recently, in which no less than 423 – i.e. nearly 20% were found to be suffering from depressive illness. Yet the incidence is probably much higher than this in actual fact, for it is authoritatively stated that general practitioners fail to recognise between 30% – 50% of their patients actually suffering from depression, by reason of the fact that a physical disorder is presented by the patient which usually diverts attention from the true cause. In other words, through the very nature of the illness causing as it does often some definite physical troubles such as headaches, stomach troubles, etc, treatment is directed to these symptoms leaving the real cause completely overlooked.

The actual symptoms shown by people with depression vary considerably, and two different people behaving in markedly different ways can both be classed as being depressed. The picture becomes even more complex when the condition is accompanied by acute anxiety or by bouts of almost forced gaiety, talkativeness and compulsive activity. However, in general depression moods may vary from slight sadness to intense despair, accompanied by a feeling of utter worthlessness.

Unfortunately, and strangely, people in this condition seldom talk of their feelings to their doctor which is a great pity. Instead they will talk of their aches and pains, their tiredness or even their loss of weight. They may even find it difficult to speak at all, yet others may seem to chatter on ceaselessly. Either may be a sign of depression.

These differences are often the result of thought difficulties. Many will complain that they are not able to think clearly, concentrate, or make decisions for themselves, although they KNOW something is amiss. Realizing their own state without seemingly being able to do anything about it affects depressives in another way. They tend to be preoccupied with themselves, and quite unable to count their blessings. Instead, they will magnify the mishaps of the past and tend to blow them up into major disasters, the whole time regarding themselves as totally to blame for these misfortunes.

This habit of distorting events to their own detriment, affects their sleep, which may already be badly disturbed by their tinnitus, and on going to bed they will usually lie awake worrying about the past, about their present state, and about that of the future. This easily sets up a vicious circle with the worry concerning their inability to sleep adding itself to all the others. And as if this is not enough, the depression itself will probably be causing early morning wakening which as all of us know is fatal to any further sleep.

When depression is accompanied by anxiety, the sufferer is usually very restless and develops a nervous way of talking. This is vastly different from the apathy of other depressives who rather tend to hide their worries from others.

Most GP's will tell you that many of their patients actually suffering from depression regard this as being something that is socially unacceptable (an outdated conception) and so they present themselves with some other complaint entirely. This is really grossly unfair on the doctors, and in the medical profession is known as 'coming with a ticket'.

Reactive Depression such as that caused by bereavement can be more long lasting than Endogenous Depression such as we have discussed. It is quite normal to express grief at the death of a loved one, and indeed to attempt to suppress such grief reactions just because they are painful or because one may feel that the dead person 'would not like me to be sad' is never helpful. In fact this attitude undoubtedly tends to prolong the period of grief.

Besides the usual reactions of distress at bereavement there are often feelings of guilt; a feeling that one should have done more for the dead person, there can also be considerable irritability and great lack of warmth towards others. People in this state often have problems in their relationships with other members of the family and with friends. They sometimes show intense feelings of anger toward doctors, hospitals or so-called 'uncaring' relatives.

On the other side of the coin with some people there may be a complete lack of any apparent signs of grief, accompanied by periods of restlessness and engaging in virtually pointless activities, such as repetitive housework and the like. In such cases as this the grieving person should be actively encouraged to let out their pent-up feelings and talk about their loss.

One theory concerning depression whether caused by illness or grief is that it probably results from an imbalance of two types of chemicals within the brain. One lifts us up. The other casts us down. Thus the effect of imbalance either way results in depression. Perfect balance is the norm.

Many people find it hard to appreciate the depths of despair that can affect a severely depressed person. We have to realise that depression is in itself no fleeting symptom. Fortunately, with the latest medications available depression can be effectively and permanently treated by your own GP in the majority of cases.

In the past, drugs for the treatment for depression have revolved around the early tranquillizers with their often horrific side effects. However the latest anti-depressants which are known as 'Second Generation Anti-depressants' give very few side effects, and with some people none at all. Additionally they are extremely effective.

This should give anyone suffering from depression every encouragement to seek medical help. However, in the use of any such drug it should be known that its action may take up to three or sometimes four weeks before it becomes even noticeable. Thus, especially with cases of depression, patience is the essence of a cure, and any drug prescribed should be taken regularly and conscientiously. A depressed person is naturally pessimistic and on finding no immediate relief can well abandon the treatment entirely. This should never be done.

With medication taken conscientiously, within four to six weeks a depressed person should start to feel their old self again, but it is recommended that the treatment should continue for a total of six months. The treatment can then be gradually withdrawn or stopped. There are no withdrawal symptoms with the latest such drugs, and above all you cannot 'get hooked' on them.

LIVING WITH DEPRESSION AND HOW YOU CAN HELP

If you are living with someone with depression, even though they are taking medication, do not expect too much too soon. It is a fairly long haul, and much patience is needed no matter how infuriatingly negative the sufferers behaviour may be.

What is most needed is your continual friendliness, come what may. Swallow your feelings and repress any possibly hurtful remarks, difficult as this may sometimes be.

You will help them considerably by encouraging them to take their medication regularly and especially encouraging them through those periods of pessimism in which they take the attitude that the medication is doing them no good.

Even if they do not respond, it is up to you to take a positive attitude – this will be remembered with gratitude later when they are well again.

Under no circumstances should you invoke them to 'Pull yourself together' nor should you suggest that they need to get away from it all and take a holiday, for you would unfortunately find that they would at this stage certainly fail to benefit from such things as holidays, for they would become even more anxious and depressed when on unfamiliar ground. Reserve such things as holidays for them until the time when they are well on the road to recovery. This will benefit everyone concerned. Just encourage them to carry on with a normal life – reassure them that they are needed and above all else . . . that they are LOVED!

Chapter Ten

Tinnitus and Stress

With the onset of Tinnitus, stress is, it would appear, almost immediately generated by this sudden alarming and overwhelming noise. The noise has been very aptly likened to a signal of pain. Again it is the old fundamental animal instinct within us all – Fight or Flight – there is no escaping it.

A regular irritating noise such as Tinnitus causes us to be constantly and rigidly mobilised for instant action, and as surely as night follows day this state of affairs will have the effect of producing certain physical disorders.

Stress drives the body to liberate hormones which stimulate its ability to Escape or Conquer. These hormones come chiefly from the pituitary and adrenal glands and they also include a considerable amount of other secretions, each with a specific target organ of the body on which they have immediate effect.

To explain a little more explicitly exactly what is meant by stress having effect upon target organs of the body, I would ask you to recall say your last visit to the dentist, perhaps your last examination day, or your wedding day, or those last few moments before you were due to go on stage. You will be in no doubt regarding the target area of the body affected in these moments of stress as you pay yet another visit to what is known in polite society as 'the little room'!

This is of course only temporary stress, continuing stress will more gradually show its effects. One's skin is a prime target, and I am sure many Tinnitus sufferers will recall unexplained rashes appearing on different parts of the body whilst under stress.

The stomach is another target organ frequently giving rise to indigestion, ulcers and so on. The digestive system is another prime target of stress and a variety of worrying conditions may be set up, yet all may well be stress-related.

Similarly the cardio-vascular system concerned with the heart and blood can give rise to quite alarming conditions under stress.

Unfortunately, the problems that beset us all in the organized community in which we live, can only very seldom be resolved quickly by some direct action, and so these stimuli lead to a state of persistent reaction and over-reaction which develop quickly into symptoms of anxiety, fear and frustration.

Such then, can be the ultimate effects of severe Tinnitus, but the extent of attention that people give to their Tinnitus can control the condition of stress quite considerably. A focus of attention on the symptom will certainly increase the sensation of the noises and so add to the stress.

Even the most well-adjusted among us will agree that the sounds of Tinnitus become much worse when one is tired or ill, or during any emotional conflict.

In addition to this, upbringing and the personality factor greatly affect the attitude of patients in regard to their Tinnitus. Too great an attention to this physical disturbance can worsen the sensations, and thus result in the noises appearing to be much worse than they actually are.

It is also strange that in most matching studies that are undertaken it is constantly being discovered that not all Tinnitus sufferers perceive the disturbance of Tinnitus in the same way, and patients having precisely the same type, frequency and degree of noise are not all equally bothered by it. In one comparison test, two sets of patients were interviewed. One set were people who were not over-disturbed by their Tinnitus and reported that they could well cope with it, and had no history of debilitating episodes. The other set were of sufferers greatly debilitated by their noises, yet it was found that in each set the actual intensity of the Tinnitus was equal.

An individual's psychological reaction to stress varies considerably, depending on the origin of the stress, one's ego, maturity and type of thinking. In so many the stress becomes overwhelming. With some the noises are a constant reminder that all is not well with them and accentuates the dread that there is no cure for their Tinnitus.

With far too many patients considerable problems occur when their Tinnitus becomes an obsession with them. Personality changes can occur with Tinnitus becoming a scapegoat with needs and conflicts being loaded on to this one symptom. Such an obsession can all too easily lead on to further neurotic behaviour, social withdrawal and problems with reality.

One Tinnitus Clinic reports that over half the patients who attend would never present themselves for help but for the presence of the coexisting stress factor which adds so much to the symptom and makes it all the more unbearable. In such cases it is fruitless and unrealistic to try to approach the Tinnitus itself in isolation. The reason for this is that the patient's fears, worries and anxieties are intermeshed and interact with the symptoms of Tinnitus in so many different ways, although the patient may be quite unaware of these factors without proper counselling.

However, this is not always easy for the counsellor, because the patient is more interested in something physical being done about the symptom, i.e. the Tinnitus itself, than with efforts to come to terms with the conflicts which may in many cases be causing it.

An expert counsellor will try to answer a patient's question by another question or turn the patient's question around so that the patient can well end up answering the question himself, but unfortunately this strategy is unhelpful in dealing with specific questions regarding the Tinnitus itself.

Stress is a strange problem with us, for example a job which is too undemanding or boring can be equally as stressful as one that involves overworking or excessive responsibility and we must always remember that the way we feel mentally or emotionally can affect the way in which our bodies react and function, and we can feel just as unwell from stress as from any physical disease.

Chapter Eleven

Main Causes of Tinnitus

NOISE TRAUMA

Loss of hearing induced by exposure to loud noise will usually bring Tinnitus with it. Exposure to such noise for a period of even ten minutes can result in temporary Tinnitus.

Provided one is not exposed to such loud noises regularly, any permanent effect still appears to be negligible. Unfortunately many people are obliged to work in noisy factories and workplaces in which they are being constantly bombarded with high noise levels. In such cases the effects cease to remain temporary and indeed within a reasonable time can cause considerable trouble.

The onset is insidious – the effect working secretly in the background until it breaks forth to betray us.

For example. A new hand arrives for work in a noisy factory. He it totally unused to the loud noise. He may have worked as a farmhand or gardener previously. Without being aware of it, by the end of the first day he may have acquired a considerable threshold shift in his hearing. Maybe a slight ringing in his ears. On the way home he may be aware that his car engine sounds particularly quiet, and when he mows the lawn that evening his mower appears to purr over the grass, much to his satisfaction.

The following day he may well discover that the slight Tinnitus he went to bed with has disappeared, and possibly without his being aware of it his hearing has partially recovered. The days which follow will not have such an apparent effect on him for as time goes on he will become accustomed to the threshold shift and therefore the factory noises become (apparently) less intense. Without being aware of it, or even acknowledging it he will gradually be acquiring some degree of hearing loss. If this goes on for a year or so he will gradually become aware of his hearing loss. He will need the television or radio with more volume, possibly to the annoyance of his family; conversation, especially in close noisy situations will become difficult; he may experience difficulty with the location of sounds. Alas the damage is done and as he reaches the evening of his life he will probably be extremely deaf, and will also probably have suffered from Tinnitus for some considerable time. This alas, is the usual sad story and should be a warning to all.

Since 1972 Codes of Practice related to hearing damage in industry have been brought out but unfortunately do not always appear to be observed. The laying down of such legislation is obviously not without its difficulties, for the reaction to noise exposure varies between one individual and another. Constant exposure to a certain level of noise can damage the hearing of one person and yet not another or affect one severely and another less.

Those noises built up of pure tones are usually more damaging than noises of broad band composition and machinery giving off a noise of a loud single note or succession of notes, particularly damaging.

Returning again to the problems of the Tinnitus sufferer it is an odd fact that certain loud noises can quite badly exacerbate the noises of Tinnitus even in those who have had Tinnitus for many years. Curiously, from the reports available, such sounds vary considerably from person to person.

The sound of loud machinery of any kind is the noise mostly complained of in this context, but other sounds such as hammering, certain musical notes, TV or radio, a sharp clap or sudden sound, very high pitched noises or over loud music are but a few of the 'triggers' that can cause this effect. Hallam et al (1984) stated that among his patients he discovered that those with binaural Tinnitus were the more likely to have their Tinnitus exacerbated by noise than those with the Tinnitus in one ear only and that 43 per cent of those whose Tinnitus appeared to be induced by loud noise found it to be worsened by other noises, against only 15 per cent of those whose hearing loss had not been associated with noise.

As will be seen, the effect of loud noises on our hearing are cumulative and in the present climate in which noise pollution even in our daily lives seems hardly to be taken seriously it is up to each individual to protect themselves as far as possible.

Even the use of lawn mowers, electric drills, chain saws and outboard motors etc. should never be undertaken without adequate ear protection.

Our ears are delicate and extremely complex organs – so complex that medical science has still much to learn about them. Just think of this. Our ears can hear sounds which are over ten billion times as loud as the very softest sounds they can detect! They analyse the sounds that we hear into frequency elements, they are noise-band and frequency analysers in addition. They are useful to us in monitoring our own speech. They tell us from which direction a sound is coming, and in addition part of them is our organ of balance. Is it not therefore only sensible that we should all protect our ears and our hearing at all costs?

DISCOS Apart from many people working in noisy environments, the tendency these days especially for the younger ones is to continue with this into their recreational activities. Most equipment at Discos and Pop Concerts is notoriously overloud, – a statement proven by the many musicians who have now gone deaf and suffer from Tinnitus. Was it not 'The Who' that later suggested they be re-named 'The What?'.

AGEING One of the main causes of Tinnitus in the elderly certainly arises from the loss of hearing due to the degeneration of the tiny hair cells of the cochlea and the thickening of the basilar membrane, the vibration of which is affected by becoming stiffer.

There is usually difficulty in hearing high pitched sounds, and although vowels can be heard reasonably well there is usually some difficulty over certain consonants, thus causing conversational problems.

OTOSCLEROSIS

I feel that no book on Tinnitus would be complete without reference to this tragically incapacitating disease which can affect us in early adulthood just at the time when all life opens before us.

It is a disease with a definite hereditary link – females are twice as liable to it as males. Since pregnancy triggers the onset in many cases it is wise for those women with a family history of early hearing loss to obtain genetic counselling before starting a family. This should in any case be done should either partner have a family history of early hearing loss.

The disease is most common between the ages of 15 to 30 and the signs and symptoms are a slow but progressive loss of hearing, Tinnitus, and the feeling that hearing is better in noisy situations than in quiet ones. Sound distortion precedes the actual deafness although this is not so severe as in the case of Meniere's Disease.

The disease causes a slow formation of abnormal spongy bone growth within the middle ear. This then prevents one of the small bones in the middle ear from vibrating. It usually unfortunately affects both ears.

The younger the patient, the more rapid one can expect the hearing loss to be. It is essential to get the matter dealt with as quickly as possible. Your GP will refer you to a specialist, for where possible surgery gives a certain benefit; otherwise the disease progresses and can become static.

MENIERE'S DISEASE

This episodic condition consists of vertigo, deafness and Tinnitus of a low pitched or rushing nature and was first reported by Dr Prosper Meniere in 1861. It had previously been thought to be a form of apoplexy or stroke. The condition is caused by an increase of pressure in the fluids of the inner ear. This fluid, known as 'endolymph hydrops' bathes both the hearing organ or cochlea and the semi-circular canals which are concerned with balance.

Dr Meniere's description of the disease is now a medical classic:

'A man, young and robust, suddenly without apparent reason experienced vertigo, nausea and vomiting. He had a state of inexpressible anguish and prostration. The face was pale and bathed in sweat as if about to faint. Often, and at the same time, the patient after seeming to stagger in a dazed state fell to the ground unable to get up. Lying on his back he could not open his eyes without his environment becoming as a whirlpool. The smallest movements of the head worsened the feeling of vertigo and nausea.'

It is reported that Meniere's Disease affects some 46 out of

100,000 and is more common with men than women. If left untreated it becomes progressively worse. There is no way of predicting an attack which can come at any time, a fact which causes considerable apprehension and worry with the sufferer for they may find themselves experiencing an attack in most embarrassing situations.

Verification of the condition is fairly complex and takes time. The usual test is one known as the 'Caloric Test' which embodies the irrigation of either ear with warm water slightly above body temperature. This, in altering the temperature of the inner ear fluids causes them to move and in watching the eye movements at this time it is possible to check on the efficiency of the balance mechanism in each ear. This helps in arranging the further management of the patient.

One important dietary factor of this condition lies in the reduction of salt intake, since this causes the retention of fluids. There is a salt substitute that can be obtained and used, both in cooking and on food.

There are two drugs which have been found especially helpful for this condition. One is Serc (Betahistine) and the other Stemetil (Prochlorperazine).

Somewhat fortunately, the Tinnitus which accompanies Meniere's Disease can very likely be masked by a suitable Tinnitus Masker and even sometimes by just a hearing aid. Most patients also find that successful drug treatment of the vertigo additionally reduces the tinnitus.

There exist a number of conditions that can closely mimic Menieres Disease and there must be a number of people under treatment for this condition that just do not have it at all.

Recently one of the members of my group, a man in his mid-fifties presented to his doctor with tinnitus and dizzy spells. He had a loss of balance and trembling in the legs. He was unable to bend down without losing his balance completely, and neither could he turn around quickly without a similar effect. He found when walking, should he look around he would find himself not walking in the same direction as would anyone in normal health.

Following a second visit to his doctor he was prescribed Serc which is the usual prescription for Menieres Disease, and certainly from the symptoms the doctor was quite right to do so. Correctly of course he should have awaited the test that has been described, but probably in the knowledge that this might not be possible to be arranged for some time, he took the obvious course.

But the Serc so upset this patient that very sensibly after 4 days he went back to the doctor who immediately took him off it, and in view of his distressed condition arranged for an ENT specialist to see him.

Throughout all this the patient's hearing was extremely good and showed up well on the hearing tests that he underwent. Following a very careful examination the ENT Specialist arrived at the conclusion that the man was not suffering from any inner ear problem at all, and that the cause was a neurological one.

Referred to the Neurological Department of his local hospital, this patient underwent various tests which included a CAT scan. This plainly indicated that he was suffering beyond doubt from what is known as Transient Ischaemic Attacks or 'TIA's'. These attacks are caused by hardening of the arteries to the brain thus resulting in deficient blood supply. Yet how near to Menieres the symptoms were?

In his case the arteries had become 'furred up' and hardened and little portions of the 'fur' together with groups of blood cells break off causing temporary blockages 'downstream'.

As readers will doubtless be aware, normally anyone with tinnitus is warned not to take aspirin as it can exacerbate the condition, but this patient has been put on a very low dose of aspirin [obviously to thin the blood] for so low a dose would be very unlikely to affect his tinnitus. He is also on Atenolol to control his blood pressure and some diuretic tablets to control liquid retention.

He is now free of all the previous symptoms and obtaining up to three days complete remission from time to time of his tinnitus.

Ear Wax (Cerumen)

Some people produce too much wax in the ears and normally go to their GP to have their ears syringed, but I have had dozens of people inform me that their tinnitus started immediately they came out of their doctor's after having their ears syringed. Why this should be is not quite clear but I always recommend

Members to ask their GP to refer them to a specialist for the Dry Method of Wax Removal. This is done with the aid of a special magnifying microscope, and a plastic or metal probe. The wax is removed by fine forceps and completed by aspiration from a suction tube attached to a small vacuum pump. I am told by those who have had this done that it is quite pleasant and only takes a short while. On the basis that it is better to be safe than sorry I do feel that anyone susceptible to tinnitus and certainly anyone with it, should use this method.

Tinnitus and the Teeth

Tinnitus can be caused by the jaw not occluding properly when it is thought that there is a connection with the small muscles at the side of the face with the ossicles of the ear. In such cases usually the teeth do not occlude properly when the jaw is closed, but much can be done by the insertion of a small plastic easily removeable correction piece which can be fitted over a few of the teeth on the side required. The problem is known as Temporomandibular Jaw Dysfunction. (For more detail please see Chapter Seventeen.)

Cervical Spondylosis

One of the main signs of the problem are crunching sounds with the movement of the neck affected by a slight misalignment among the seven small bones at the top of the spine. Following X-rays of the neck it is often possible for a Chiropractor to be of help. If the symptoms are minor they will usually respond well to treatment, but subside slowly. Many experts advise sleeping without a pillow, and sometimes a 'Thomas Collar' of soft fabric will help.

Prescribed Drugs

Drugs prescribed by your doctor can so often prove to be ototoxic. Those that affect the auditory system fall into two distinct groups – those that can cause either temporary or permanent loss of hearing and are liable to give rise to Tinnitus as a secondary condition, or those that can actually cause Tinnitus without being associated with hearing loss.

This is why it is so essential that anyone with Tinnitus should tell their doctor that they have this problem preferably at the time that any drug is prescribed for them no matter for what purpose. Remember your doctor is there to help you.

Stress

The stress which so often can cause Tinnitus and at the same time be generated by the actual onset of the noises is dealt with fully in Chapter Ten.

Accident

Certain types of accident, especially those involving the head can cause Tinnitus. A 'whiplash' car accident, a sudden sports strain, a bad fall or even when the neck itself becomes misaligned due to incorrect posture – all these things can result in Tinnitus, many of them lying in the domain of the Chiropractor.

Chapter Twelve

Self Help

Judging from various reports of studies made over the last few years it appears that some 60% of Tinnitus sufferers, when first experiencing the condition, received no help whatever. This is indeed a sad state of affairs, for it is just at this time when a sufferer needs all the help available by way of empathy and understanding, guidance over depression, and general easing of the anxiety experienced by the onset of this really quite alarming symptom.

It is at this stage that the joining of a Tinnitus Self-Help Group can mean so much, enabling one to talk with other sufferers, some of whom have possibly had Tinnitus for years and have, in their own way, learned to cope with it.

Just to talk with someone who understands can do so much to relieve the fear and anxiety which usually accompanies the condition, especially at the outset. Associating with others will also avoid the possibility of becoming insular, which is so often the lot of many sufferers, especially those who live alone.

Most experts agree that any counselling undertaken within a Self-Help Group should be by a person who also has Tinnitus. This rather sets the condition apart from the usual ills wherein one seeks the advice of someone with a medical degree.

The aims of such Groups have now become almost universal: To extend mutual support, help and comfort to other members. To provide and discuss the latest information on Tinnitus Research and coping strategies. To hold regular meetings at which expert Guest Speakers are invited. To provide a Telephone Helpline, and to engage in social activities wherever possible.

Such Groups are normally run on a non-profit basis, administration being unpaid. A Committee comprising Chairman, Secretary and Treasurer is appointed from the membership usually acting on a yearly basis. Committee meetings should be held and minutes drawn up. An annual general meeting enables Members to vote regarding the appointment of the Committee for the coming year.

Such a Group enables those with Tinnitus to meet in a mutually supportive and non-threatening atmosphere, and to share experiences and coping strategies. Hope is instilled by the mere interaction with others, especially from those who have passed through the first difficult phase.

A monthly Newsletter is usually sent to each Member containing all the latest information pertaining to the Group with news of any latest research, and the date of the next meeting. A partner or friend is normally welcomed to accompany any member to meetings for all are fully aware of the effects of Tinnitus on relationships.

There can be no finer environment for any Tinnitus sufferer than the meetings of Self-Help Groups. There they find themselves among people with a genuine interest in each other and who understand each other's problems. They know that despite a certain amount of sympathy from others, including partners, friends, doctors and so on, these people just cannot really understand precisely what life can be like with a constant noise in the head or ears, day after day without respite.

The precise benefit that members obtain from a Self-Help Group is rather difficult to define, for it lies in the interaction of many things, including the comradeship induced by the mutual sharing of a problem, the feeling of helpful support, and the gaining of knowledge over a matter which for so many is currently completely spoiling the quality of their lives.

It is so helpful to be able to unburden one's feelings to someone with the same difficulties in a non-threatening atmosphere so unlike that of a normal clinical environment. Because they have been assured that the normal medical channels can help them but little, they find comfort in the lectures, friendly talks, and informative newsletters which every good Self-Help Group provides. They join with the others in exploring the possibilities of various ways of reducing stress, anxiety, depression, insomnia and so on that are all too often the associated symptoms of this condition.

They are encouraged to help other sufferers, and belonging to such a Group gives them the added feeling of being useful and part of a number of other people who are at least trying to do something about their mutual problems. They meet others who are far worse off than themselves, and yet still manage to cope. All of this is good for them.

This attitude gives the feeling of having more control over their own lives by actually joining those who are trying to exert some influence for good, and by feeling part of it. All this engenders a psychological adjustment to their own problems – the feeling that they are not at the mercy of some force against which they feel helpless; that no longer are they passively accepting their problems, but trying to do something about them.

In the absence of any orthodox medical help, provided one is not expecting too much from them, it is only natural and right that people should wish to explore the possibilities of help from other sources. Thus we find considerable interest within these Groups, and indeed with Tinnitus sufferers generally in the exploration of such disciplines as Acupuncture – Biofeedback – Homeopathy – Yoga – Auricular Therapy – Chiropractic – Reflexology and any available Relaxation Therapies.

I have many times witnessed varying degrees of alleviation from one or other of these, especially with the associated symptoms of tinnitus such as depression, anxiety, insomnia and the like. Perhaps the mere fact of trying something of this nature has in itself a therapeutic effect. I do feel that every Group should encourage speakers on these subjects no matter how removed from tinnitus the discipline may appear to be.

It is also vitally important that as much correct information as possible on the subject of tinnitus should be given at Group Meetings, and in their Newsletters, and this is why it is so essential that the Group be led by a person with as much knowledge of the subject as possible, together with experience in counselling.

It is also important and helpful to educate those with tinnitus as to the considerable physical complexities of the symptom and the reasons why it is difficult to discover any simple means of alleviating or controlling it. Far too many who have been given the 'learn to live with it' advice from their GP seem full of resentment and even bitter over the way they have been treated and are overtly antagonistic toward the medical profession in general. One cannot help feeling that this is grossly unfair to the doctors.

Far too many people with tinnitus find themselves concentrating on the noises yet refraining from talking about it. This is certainly not good, for such concentration on the tinnitus can often make it appear much worse than it actually is.

SELF HELP HINTS

The following are a few useful suggestions and guide-lines, each based on either medical or anecdotal evidence which many people with Tinnitus have found helpful. Since there is such a wide variety of reasons for the condition, that which helps one person may well not help another. It should be mentioned that in Tinnitus Management it is found that most people experience a certain amount of alleviation anyway by trying to help themselves in this way (placebo effect?) and in any case certainly no harm can be done by following any of the suggestions put forward.

ASPIRIN not only exacerbates Tinnitus but can cause it as well. If you find an analgesic necessary, take something like Paracetamol.

ANXIETY and STRESS will always make Tinnitus appear to be much worse, for the auditory system of a person with tinnitus is usually fairly tense in any case.

ALCOHOL which is popularly regarded as a stimulant is in fact a sedative. Some argue that in strict moderation it helps them to relax but experts point out that alcohol is universally recognised as a powerful ear-damaging agent especially when used in excess, and can in certain circumstances actually cause tinnitus.

CAFFEINE acts as a stimulant to the central nervous system and is present in considerable quantity in ordinary tea and coffee. Fortunately both tea and coffee are now available in decaffeinated forms in which the caffeine content has been cut to a minimum. It is far better to use these at all times.

COCOA also chocolate and chocolate drinks alas all contain considerable amounts of caffeine and are best avoided.

FATIGUE is something everyone with tinnitus should try to avoid. It is a known fact that the noises are always at their worst when we are tired. More careful planning of one's day can help tremendously.

GLUCOSE will be found helpful in many cases for dealing with 'the morning roar' i.e. the sensation that the tinnitus is much louder on awakening. This is thought to be due to a lowering of one's blood sugar during sleep, and many find a glass of Lucozade drink or a couple of Glucose tablets are very effective in reducing the sound to its normal level. (Not for diabetics of course).

PILLOW HEIGHT is something every person with tinnitus should experiment over. Raising the head even with three pillows can often help by relieving any possible congestion of blood in the auditory system. Also of help with neck problems.

HEAVY MEALS will often be found to increase the intensity of one's tinnitus. Regular small meals are advised.

SALT INTAKE is important for those with tinnitus and the restriction of the intake of salt has been found to create considerable relief for many people. In the case of Meniere's Disease it is essential. Strict followers of the no salt regime also limit their fluid intake to 2½ pints a day and avoid such things as bacon, cheese, salted butter, ham, kippers, marmite etc. and it should be noted that frozen food with 'oven ready' classification (i.e. complete meals only requiring heating) should be avoided if possible if a strict sodium-free diet is the aim.

SMOKING is certainly OUT! Tobacco smoke in any form is known to be bad for tinnitus, even 'passive smoking' i.e. the inhalation in a smoky environment can affect the condition.

Chapter Thirteen

Problems of Sound Location

Accurate knowledge concerning any difficulties which puzzle us can help tremendously by diminishing the anxiety that so many experience concerning certain problems associated with their Tinnitus. The unknown is always frightening, and with Tinnitus our personal attitude to the problem is all-important.

So many Tinnitus sufferers refer to the difficulties they experience in the location of sounds, and ask why this should be, appearing to feel that they are probably the only people to have this particular problem; as do many others who refer to the great difficulty they have in holding a conversation in crowded company. This causes them to avoid such situations and thereby seriously affects the quality of life by their becoming somewhat isolated.

In the first case, the sort of situation that usually occurs is for example when one calls out to someone in the house who answers them, but they are quite unable to locate the direction of the other person's voice and may well start to walk in the opposite direction in order to try to contact them. This situation is not helped when they call out 'Where are you?' and the other person answers 'In here!' – leaving them as fogged as ever. Quite a number of people, especially the more elderly are particularly concerned over this problem, for quite rightly they feel it could be dangerous in certain situations; for example in crossing the road when the direction of a speeding vehicle could be so easily misjudged.

The second case is of course bound up with the same problem and results in a person being unable to separate wanted sound (i.e. the voice of the person to whom they are talking) from the unwanted sound or seeming myriad of voices of others around them.

To appreciate the reasons behind this difficulty we must understand that the Pinna or external part of the ear acts as a kind of funnel in the reception of sound. A sound comes to us through the air, but remember that the final destination of that sound is our cochlea which is filled with fluid. It will readily be understood that the resistance therefore to a sound wave coming to us through the air is vastly different to the resistance of that same sound wave when passing into the fluid-filled cochlea.

It is therefore necessary for the mechanism of our ear to equalise the fairly low resistance of sound through air so that it matches the required resistance of sound to the cochlea.

The convoluted shape of the pinna has the effect of breaking up certain frequencies between the various sound paths entering the ear canal. With normal hearing these changes alter according to the differing directions from which the sound is coming, and thus accurately inform us of the direction of that sound. Our other ear reinforces this information by reason of its differing position in the path of the sound wave. Therefore sound localisation is extremely difficult where there is a greater loss of hearing in one of the ears compared with the other, or deafness in one ear with the association of tinnitus. The reason it is so difficult to locate the actual direction of sounds is because these have not been filtered by the pinna, nor have they been filtered subsequently by other parts of the auditory system. The ear canal not only protects the middle and inner ear, but acts as a resonator rather like an organ pipe, and this further helps in the matching or the resistance between that of air and the fluid of the cochlea.

The middle ear also acts as yet another transformer of the resistance between air and the needs of the cochlea. Since this action is under the control of certain small muscles it is capable of closing down quickly during loud sounds, and opening up in quieter moments in order to pick up the quieter sounds, this being the natural way of protecting the delicate cochlea.

As a simplification of all this, let us imagine a sound coming from the end of the room in which you are reading this. The Pinna of your ear receives that sound through the air, but in order for you to hear this sound correctly it has to be filtered by the Pinna of your ear, then the ear canal, then the middle ear, and then through the fluid of your cochlea.

Thus several things have to occur. The Pinna of your ear by its various convolutions causes subtle changes in the actual frequencies of the sound. These changes alter according to the direction from which the sound is coming and in normal hearing the other ear would reinforce this information by its differing position in relation to the source of the sound.

However, in the case of a person with loss of hearing in one ear or being more deaf in one ear than the other, it does not unfortunately work like this. They have lost the 'stereo effect' which gives a person with normal hearing the sense of direction from which any sound is coming.

Additionally, in noisy surroundings or company, the Pinna of the normal ear also helps us to separate sound that is wanted, from that which is not. This explains the other difficulty that so many experience which has become known as 'The Cocktail Party Effect' in which one becomes particularly unable to 'home in' on the person to whom you are talking, due to all the other noises around you.

It is an unfortunate fact of life that many of the loudspeakers used in the amplification of sound in such venues as Theatres and Discos, have their Resonance Peaks in the very same frequency region of high sensitivity which we use for speech, and so it can easily be understood why there is such a high risk of damage to the hearing by loud noises in this region under these conditions, so easily causing eventual deafness with probable Tinnitus.

So many people feel that they are alone with these difficulties, but I would want them to know that such problems are experienced by practically everyone with hearing loss of the type mentioned. Provided we are aware of it, understand the reasons behind it, and extend great care especially in those situations such as when in traffic when it can be dangerous, then we can cope with it accordingly.

Ironically, in actual fact an old fashioned ear trumpet really had considerable advantage over the modern electronic hearing aid in one respect. The modern aid amplifies all the unwanted and irrelevant sound as well as the voice the owner wishes to hear, whereas the ear trumpet could be so directed as to catch only the voice or other sound that the person wanted to hear. But at least the hearing aid can give warning of approaching traffic!

Chapter Fourteen
Tinnitus Research

Constant enquiries are being made as to precisely what type of research goes on in the quest for Tinnitus alleviation. Unfortunately, most avenues of research in this context end in a complete cul de sac, and it is back again to square one, for Tinnitus is a most devious problem.

THE GINGKO TREE

In the *Sunday Times* dated August 10th 1986 an article appeared which was at the time of the greatest interest to all with Tinnitus. It was headlined 'Hearing turns over a new leaf' and read:

'Failing hearing can be revived dramatically by an extract from the prehistoric Gingko Tree. The extract can also banish Tinnitus or ringing in the ears. Dr Sprenger of Germany who has been studying the extract's effect, reported earlier this year on significant improvements in thirty-five out of fifty-nine patients treated with the gingko extract, as well as the vanishing of Tinnitus in twelve out of thirty-three patients. Taken orally as either drops or tablets the extract is ideal for people whose hearing has been damaged by loud noises. There appears to be no effect whatever on normal cells, but regeneration is triggered in damaged cells, particularly the so-called 'hair cells' inside the spiral organ of the inner ear'.

This sounded absolutely wonderful! Could this be the very break-through in research that every Tinnitus sufferer had hoped for?

There was quite a stir at the British Tinnitus Association, and with a similar report appearing in The Daily Telegraph, Dr Jonathan Hazell the Consultant Neuro-Otologist at the RNID in London who is regarded as the pioneer in Tinnitus research in Britain wrote that to say the least the facts had been somewhat exaggerated; nevertheless any reports of medical treatment helping those with Tinnitus or hearing loss must be taken seriously.

However, he noted that the tests were uncontrolled, and that the extract's effects were not compared by the administration of placebos to some of those patients taking part in the test, which is usually done. Also this paper stated that of the thirty-two patients suffering from Tinnitus 30% were said to have had a disappearance of their Tinnitus at the end of the test; but in 50% of these patients there had been no change in the symptom at all. He took pains to point out that this hardly justified the wording of the report that stated 'in most cases Tinnitus was eliminated'. Also any reported changes in hearing were quite small, and then only at certain frequencies, yet the paper reports said 'one in four regained their hearing in full'.

He summed up by saying 'It is unlikely that any single substance will reverse the process of degenerative change which is the cause of most sensory hearing impairment and the cause of Tinnitus'.

At this stage Dr Ross Coles, Deputy Director of the Institute of Hearing Research at the University of Nottingham stepped in, and in the magazine "The Soundbarrier" of December 1986 he wrote:

'On our own volition and with the help of the Company' (there was by now a German Company producing this extract under the name Gingko Biloba Extract) 'we are intending to undertake a trial of GBE in patients with hearing impairment and Tinnitus. This depends on obtaining permission from the DHSS as this product has not yet been licensed in Great Britain.

The trial will be in two stages. The first will be a three months open trial, explaining to patients that GBE is totally unproven. If we obtain any encouraging reports we will go on to a formal clinical trial'.

Alas, with the publication of his report later the findings were most disappointing, for of twenty-one patients, eleven reported no change whatever in their Tinnitus. As to hearing, two of the patients started with total deafness and this remained unchanged. Four reported that their Tinnitus was slightly less, although in three of these cases it was known that the Tinnitus reduction was really caused by a lessening of certain stresses in these patients' lives. Five of the patients reported that their Tinnitus was even worse, and during the course of the study ten patients complained of side-effects.

Dr Coles completed his report by adding 'Although I do not feel that I could recommend GBE to a patient of mine, I would not attempt to dissuade anyone who wanted to try it from doing so. However, I understand that GBE will not be available in this country, and therefore supplies would only be possible from abroad. It is however available in a homeopathic potency of 6 from a firm in Derbyshire.'

As I write this, great expectations are centred on a newly started project in Research at The Ferens Institute, Middlesex Hospital, under Dr Jonathan Hazell FRCS who is the Consultant Neuro-Otologist to the RNID and regarded as the leading pioneer in Tinnitus Research in this country.

The project aims to increase understanding of the ways in which the efferent nerves running from the brain to the cochlea or inner ear might influence the activity of the sensory hair cells of the cochlea.

These cells are already known to play a fundamental role in the normal hearing process, converting the sound vibrations entering the ear into electrical impulses which are, in turn, sent via the auditory nerve to the brain.

It has been established that stimulation of the efferent nerves influences the physical activity of the outer hair cells and the pattern of signals passing from the inner hair cells up the auditory nerve.

It is now planned to use a new computerised system to test two hypotheses: that the efferent system is involved in generating some forms of tinnitus and that it might alter the perception of tinnitus, explaining why tinnitus varies so frequently with stress, exercise and other changes in an individual's condition.

Tinnitus and non-tinnitus groups will be tested using acoustic stimulation of the opposite ear to activate the efferent system. The following will be investigated:

(1) Whether altering the level of excitation of the efferent system results in modification of any kind of tinnitus perception.

(2) Whether increased or reduced activity of the efferent system influences the hearing threshold, frequency discrimination and psychoacoustical tuning curves, particularly in the region of the tinnitus frequency.

(3) Whether it is possible to relate efferent activity to variability of Brain Stem Evoked Responses in tinnitus and non-tinnitus subjects.

It is heartening to be informed that promising results have already been obtained from preliminary work on the test system.

The information gathered will have a direct bearing on the development of new theories for treating tinnitus. For example, it may become possible, in appropriate cases, to prescribe drugs which will alter efferent activity, reducing the overall level of tinnitus or limiting the disturbing fluctuations in tinnitus which so many sufferers experience.

The Norfolk Tinnitus Society has been proud to make several helpful donations to this project through Sponsored Walks and other activities, and intend to continue to do so.

It is understood that clinical trials are planned to be undertaken by Researchers at the University of Keele and Clinicians at the North Staffordshire Hospital complex to assess the effectiveness of Amiloride in tinnitus treatment.

They also wish to evaluate the effectiveness of Serc, a drug currently prescribed by some ENT Specialists, usually in cases where tinnitus is part of Meniere's syndrome.

The sensory hair cells of the inner ear or cochlea are known to play a fundamental role in the normal hearing process, converting the sound vibrations entering the ear into electrical impulses which are, in turn, sent via the auditory nerve to the brain. These cells almost certainly play an important role in tinnitus.

Amiloride has been shown to block channels activated by glutamate, a neurotransmitter thought to be essential for the correct functioning of the synapse (contact) between hair cells and the auditory nerve. There is also physiological and anatomical evidence of amiloride-binding sites in the hair cells.

By acting on the hair cells and this cell/nerve synapse, amiloride may be capable of reducing the spontaneous firing rate of auditory nerve fibres and hence the sensation of tinnitus.

But tinnitus is notoriously difficult to investigate and a valid drug trial would have to be very carefully designed. A feasibility study is therefore proposed in the first instance. This would include relevant searches of scientific and medical literature; discussions with other clinicians and researchers into tinnitus; the development of methods of assessing tinnitus and patients' attitudes to it; examination of patient records; the design of an appropriate trial and the securing of Ethical Committee approval.

Chapter Fifteen
Aspects of Tinnitus

Tinnitus matching, i.e. duplicating the pitch and intensity of a person's tinnitus is usually done by means of a tinnitus synthesizer. This is able to produce a tinnitus sound of one tone, two tones, noise bands or a combination of tones including a noise band.

With its fully adjustable range of frequencies it is ideal for the purpose of matching the sound being heard by the patient. It is reported that a perfectly matched sound played into the ear of an affected person will blend so well with the tinnitus that the hearer cannot discriminate between the two. But perfect matching is often difficult to achieve and especially with the more complicated sounds. So often 'octave confusion' can arise for example and a tonal sound of 440 Hz be mistaken for one of 880 Hz.

In the matching process there is a certain amount of comfort to the patient by the mere fact that the noise is at least now apparently understood. By means of the synthesizer the tinnitus may be projected so that his relatives too can hear it, proving that the patient has not imagined the condition, thus others will have a better understanding of the problem.

Tinnitus is a very devious condition, for it need not have a specific site of origin. It can be produced from many locations along the auditory chain from the tympanic membrane, cochlea, connecting nerves and the various nerve centres. Indeed, it may not be coming from the auditory system at all. Furthermore it is not a single condition with a single cause to it.

A NEUROLOGICAL STUDY OF TINNITUS

A neurological study of 121 patients suffering from subjective tinnitus was undertaken in America. The object being to try to discover the actual cause of the symptom. The tinnitus was regarded as 'chronic' (i.e. lingering or lasting – as opposed to 'acute') if the sufferer had experienced it for over a month and it did not seem to be improving spontaneously.

Each patient was required to agree to a neurological and a neuro-otological evaluation. This group was composed of the first 121 patients complaining of tinnitus at the State University Hospital of New York.

The average length of time that each patient had endured tinnitus was around twelve months. However, one had suffered tinnitus for sixty years.The ages ranged from 19 to 87 resulting in an average age of 55. Sixty-five were women and fifty-six were men.

In 36 of these patients tinnitus was the sole difficulty complained of. With 48 patients it was the principal complaint, but in 17 it formed an incidental symptom which was regarded as less bothersome than some other complaints that they had.

Patients were tested for hypertension (high blood pressure); thyrotoxicsis (excessive production of thyroid gland hormone); diabetes mellitus, and hyperlipidemia. Also a full history of drugs and other medications was obtained from each patient with particular attention being paid to those drugs often associated with tinnitus.

Regarding the neurological causes of tinnitus in this group it was found that 6 were through head injury; 4 through brainstem degeneration; and 3 through sound damage. It was also found that 26 of the 121 patients with chronic tinnitus certainly had neurological disease which was regarded as the most probable cause of the symptom.

63 of the patients had totally unexplained tinnitus.
28 of them had either epilepsy, Parkinson's disease or migraine.
15 had psychiatric problems quite unrelated to tinnitus.
11 had hypertension.
2 had diabetes mellitus.
1 had thyroid disease.

Those suffering from hypertension obtained considerable relief from their tinnitus by anti-hypertensive medication.

In summing up this test; it was stated that chronic tinnitus can develop through many problems quite outside the ear. Acoustic injury through loud noise; otosclerosis (new bone formation within the inner ear); Menieres Disease, and ear infections. But it was added that medical and neurological problems may well cause tinnitus to develop. Diabetes mellitus, thyroid disease, drug reaction, poisons and various allergies were all implicated as were vascular tumours in or overlying the brain; meningitis, strokes, contusions and multiple sclerosis. Additionally pressure on the auditory nerve can by itself cause tinnitus.

ATTITUDES

Attitudes to Tinnitus vary considerably – from feelings of mild irritation to strong suicidal desires. The range of attitude is usually closely connected with a person's ability to cope with the intrusion of the symptom. It has also much to do with their personal defence structure, a number of social factors, the degree of severity of the tinnitus and a number of otological problems should these exist.

The arrival of Tinnitus invariably causes excessive anxiety, feelings of depression, a degree of fear regarding the cause, disturbance of sleep patterns and a certain degree of general debility.

An interesting study was made in America by House based on 150 tinnitus patients referred by reason of their having described their Tinnitus as a serious problem. Half reported their Tinnitus as severe and unrelenting. Some had been on various medications, had used acupuncture or hypnosis, and others had sought and used every other known treatment option but all without result.

Many of them had begged their physicians to do whatever was necessary to stop the noises even to the extent of receiving surgical treatment that would completely destroy their hearing provided it stopped the Tinnitus. Some reported that they were severely incapacitated by the noises in their head, others said that it was seriously restricting their activities and social contacts and destroying the whole quality of their lives.

Throughout this particular study it was found that those patients with very disturbing Tinnitus fell generally into three psychological categories:

Depressive reaction
Hysterical conversion reactions
Schizoid features & character disturbances

Of the 150 patients, 132 of them were referred and tested by a Psychologist. 48 of them fell into the depressive reaction range. 54 into the Hysterical conversion reaction group and 30 were of borderline category.

In the programme of treatment which followed, those in the depressive reaction group gained the most benefit. They looked upon their Tinnitus as their most important problem. They received special attention in the relief of their depression and with the alleviation of the depression came a certain alleviation of their Tinnitus.

As regards the conversion reaction patients, although treatment yielded a certain amount of success here, there was certainly not as much improvement as that attained by the depressive reaction group. The main defences of this group were denial and repression. Low psychological insight and limited emotional maturity were also reported.

This type of sufferer seems to regard their Tinnitus as purely physical in nature causing them to strongly resist any psychological interpretation. Psychotherapy was however acceptable to some of these patients later.

The other group – the 'borderline patients' experienced considerable difficulty with the treatment. The majority of them failed entirely to complete the training in Biofeedback and reacted badly with psychotherapy. Psychologically they were all regarded as demonstrating schizoid personality features. All were found to be of a rather solitary nature, somewhat retiring, introspective and unemotional.

In evaluating this study it was felt that those patients who are the most seriously disturbed and affected by their Tinnitus are certainly the most likely to become depressive. They regard their Tinnitus as entirely physical. They have a certain obsession with bodily functions. It was even found that Biofeedback training was too threatening for some of them.

Resulting in the treatment given in this particular study some 80% of the 132 patients interviewed and tested were able to report varying degrees of reduction in the intensity of their

Tinnitus with better patterns of sleep, less medication required, a general increase in the feelings of well-being, and a better attitude toward themselves.

Even as the treatment continued it was apparent that there were encouraging changes in attitude with a number of patients reporting that they were now regarding the problem of Tinnitus as one they felt they could live with. A further feature was obviously relief from obsession with their Tinnitus which had previously been such a marked feature of their difficulties.

When considering attitudes relating to tinnitus it seems only right that the attitudes of certain experts and writers on this subject should also be examined. For example one 'expert' states that he feels some short method of counselling is all that is necessary to alleviate the distress caused by tinnitus in most sufferers. This appears to be a rather wild and inaccurate statement to make.

A certain amount of sympathy must of course be extended to doctors and others when confronted with tinnitus. They are fully aware that there is no general cure and that they are helping but little to reach for the prescription pad. But to decry in any way the importance of this debilitating condition by reason of the fact that they are unable to do very much about it is to say the least unhelpful.

Fortunately this dismissive attitude is now fairly rare among members of the medical profession, possibly due to the increased publicity and information now surrounding tinnitus.

On the other side of the coin the fault can certainly sometimes lie with the patient. Often a person will focus on their tinnitus when in reality they are seeking help for some deep psychological problem.

SPONTANEOUS OTOACOUSTIC EMISSIONS (OAE's)

Emissions of sound are detectable in the ear canal of many of us, and the general impression is that these sounds have their origin in the cochlea.

Despite these emissions being fairly common in human beings, they have also been found in such animals as guinea pigs, chinchillas and cats. There exists one extraordinary report of very intense Otoacoustic Emissions (OAE's) in both ears of a young dog. In fact it has been reported that this instance is the most intense ever measured for any species.

The dog in question was an American Eskimo dog which was only five months old when first brought to the attention of a Veterinary Surgeon. The owners complained that noises of a continuous nature were emanating from both its ears. Tests proved that the right ear produced an intense narrow-band sound of around 9060 Hz. The centre frequency of this sound was somewhere between the range of 8915 Hz to 9180 Hz.

The emission from the left ear was of a more complex nature with the four main frequencies around 9450–10,000–1042 and 10,950 Hz. The width of the bands in each component were almost identical with that of the right ear. The conclusions gained from this test with the dog caused the experts who carried out tests to arrive at the hypothesis that OAE's must have their origin in or near the organ of Corti adjacent to regions of outer hair cell loss. They state that most certainly the data from the right ear of the dog was consistent with this suggestion.

Curiously, those emissions which can be picked up by a super sensitive microphone in some human ears are not usually heard by their possessors. In those cases in which it is possible to pick up several emissions from the same ear, the owners are often only aware of just one.

Yet in an experiment, four out of ten sufferers were discovered to be hearing the same tonal sound in their tinnitus as that of their OAE. It is therefore felt that there must be some correlation between the sounds of tinnitus and OAE's and it is interesting to note that; during tests for pitch matching both the tinnitus itself and the OAE can be wiped out by the adjustment of the external sound, and also that alterations in air pressure in the outer canal of the ear will cause both tinnitus sound and OAE to rise correspondingly. However, the tonal content of tinnitus itself is not so noisy and rough as that of OAE's which does rather lead one to feel that very possibly they are noise bands.

RECRUITMENT

Many people with Tinnitus will also be found to suffer from this phenomenon of severe loudness discomfort and up until fairly recently the experts felt that this could not be helped by masking therapy. However, modern research has revealed that

fluctuations in the electrical paths of the mechanism of the inner ear.

It is an unfortunate fact that any Tinnitus of an irregular type such as this can become more irritating and debilitating than that of a constant noise. In such cases it has been found that Masking is often most helpful, for it tends to fill in the fluctuating sounds and make the condition less irritating.

GAZE-EVOKED TINNITUS

The incidence of this type of Tinnitus is unknown, but one assumes it is fairly rare. I have recently been reading the histories of two typical cases which readers may find of interest.

The first concerns a woman of fifty who was in good health but suffering from a loss of hearing. Examination revealed that she had a small tumour covering some of the cranial nerves, for which she underwent an operation. Following this she discovered she was completely unable to hear in her left ear, and furthermore tended to fall to the left.

During the following year she suddenly became aware of sounds that appeared to originate, so she said from behind her left eye. She described these sounds as a buzzing or bleeping noise occurring whenever she looked to the right or the left. In looking straight ahead it was not noticeable. She reported four differing sounds. One for each horizontal and vertical direction of her gaze.

Following further examination it was found that she experienced exactly the same tone on gazing upwards whether to the left or right and her down gaze resulted in her hearing the same tone. This tone would remain indefinitely the whole while she held her gaze in that particular direction.

Another case history of this unusual type of Tinnitus was in a man of fifty-nine suffering from an acoustic neuroma which involved the 5th 7th and 8th nerves. Following surgery for this he discovered that when moving his eyes to the right he saw three bright horizontal lines and heard a high pitched sound in his right ear.

The reasons behind this extraordinary phenomenon are said not yet to be fully understood, but some experts feel that it is caused by neural sprouting from an adjacent nerve following damage of the vestibulo-cochlea nerve which results in connections occurring between the cochlear pathways and the neural integrator for eye movements.

TINNITUS AND PRE-MENSTRUAL TENSION (PMT)

Pre-menstrual Tension affects some half of all women at some time – some very frequently. The peak incidence is to be found between the ages of 25 and 40 with symptoms usually appearing from seven to fourteen days prior to a period.

Some of the main symptoms are water retention, a tired bloated feeling and emotional tension. Sufferers from migraine often get their worst attacks during this time.

The causes are alterations in the circulating levels of hormones, especially oestrogen and progesterone. This causes a retention of sodium in the bloodstream with oedema (abnormal infiltration of tissues with fluid). Since this oedema also affects the tissues of the brain as well as the body it is easy to understand why this can aggravate some forms of Tinnitus if it causes increased pressure in the inner ear – imitating a Meniere's-like condition. This is the reason behind many women with certain types of Tinnitus reporting an increase in the severity at these times.

Tranquilisers and sedatives are rarely supplied these days. Diuretics are certainly useful, as are drugs which antagonize the effects of oestrogen. Supplements of vitamin B6 (Pyridoxine) can also be effective.

As to diet during these phases, it certainly helps to reduce salt intake, and some doctors prescribe vitamin B6 together with extra calcium.

It will be obvious that any woman with Tinnitus who is liable to PMT has at these certain times a double burden to bear involving increased irritability, emotional instability and fluctuations in sex drive.

All these symptoms can cause considerable marital problems especially when they exacerbate the depression so often already present through Tinnitus.

PMT is sometimes caused by a disorder associated with relative progesterone deficiency. In such cases many women can be helped by progesterone, or by alteration of the hormonal changes of the menstrual cycle. Expert guidance on these matters can often help considerably.

TINNITUS AND BLOOD PRESSURE

Hypertension, or high blood pressure is well known to be associated with Tinnitus, for alterations of the supply of blood to the inner ear can considerably influence the condition. Tinnitus is also thought to be associated with hardening of the arteries, a condition so often a part of the aging process. Calcium deposits itself on the walls of the arteries which can become thickened as a result of long term high blood pressure; and as we all know high blood pressure is one of the main causes of strokes, an important factor in heart attacks and kidney failure.

There are two medical terms that sound remarkably similar yet which refer to widely differing conditions. One is Hypertension and the other Hypotension. The first relates to HIGH blood pressure and the second to LOW blood pressure.

We are all familiar with having our blood pressure checked at the doctor's by means of an instrument known as a Sphygmomanometer with a flexible strap around our arm which is slowly inflated tightly in order to constrict the blood flow.

There are two readings to be observed. The top one is known as the Systolic Reading which as the heart beats records the pressure of blood against the walls of the arteries. The lower reading known as the Diastolic Reading indicates the lower pressure between the beats of the heart during which time the artery walls are relaxed.

The usual readings for the average healthy adult are 120/80 (or perhaps lower). With persons over the mid-fifties these readings can be slightly higher without causing any undue alarm. However, should a Diastolic Reading give above 105 and stay there throughout several subsequent checks, this indicates that we are approaching the 'danger zone' – i.e. indications of Hypertension.

A high reading will normally result in most doctors recommending a low-salt diet, banning the use of salt in both cooking and at meal times, together with the strict avoidance of any salty ready-made foods etc.

Some experts however, challenge this idea, claiming that Hypertension has numerous causes in addition to too much salt, pointing to too much renin (a mixture of complex organic substances that regulate blood pressure) or a combination of both these causes; sometimes, but very rarely, pointing to kidney or adrenal problems.

Most members of the medical profession are in agreement in strongly advising the cutting down of the consumption of both tea and coffee (caffeine) and especially tobacco and alcohol. In addition advice concerning the avoidance of obesity and encouragement to exercise regularly will usually be given.

In the course of living, our blood pressure jumps quite naturally up and down many times a day. This depends on our feelings and what we are doing at the time. A person with high blood pressure shows even greater 'swings' of pressure in this respect.

The circumstances under which these alterations of pressure occur are rather interesting. For example, if you are talking to your Boss your blood pressure will rise dramatically. Just as it will if you are speaking to an attractive member of the opposite sex. The same thing happens when you read anything exciting or disturbing.

Fortunately it is possible to control one's blood pressure by relaxation Techniques, but these have to be worked at and taken very seriously to produce results for you.

Most of these techniques embody five elementary disciplines:

1. Obtaining a quiet environment
2. A comfortable position; sitting or lying
3. Completely controlled muscular relaxation
4. Careful concentration on breathing
5. Clearing the mind of all thought

The most convenient and pleasurable way to undertake Relaxation is to either sit or lie (preferable) listening to one of the many special Relaxation Tapes that are available on either a tape recorder or better still a personal stereo such as a Walkman which is inaudible to anyone else. The volume of either should be as low as you can effectively use it.

Now what happens when you do this?

By relaxing both the mind and the body we cause precisely the same effect to occur as that of any of the blood pressure pills, and additionally your blood pressure stays lower in exactly the same way as it would with such a pill well after you have ceased to relax, and again entered the stresses of daily life.

It is a verified fact that Hypertension can be reduced by as much as 20% with many people merely by watching the flow of water in a brook or stream, stroking and talking to a pet, or watching tropical fish in a fish tank.

In those cases where people reach the 'danger zone' modern drug therapy is reputed to be remarkably effective. The best therapy is known as 'stepped care' in which the very mildest drug in the lowest dosage is first given. This may well be a diuretic which has the effect of lowering the pressure by ridding the body of excess fluid and salt. If this does not work, then the next step is the use of a drug to block or inhibit the stimulation of the sympathetic nervous system which causes the heart to work harder. For those few patients for whom the pressure still remains too high, the third step is that of a vasodilator which dilates narrow blood vessels.

It will thus readily be seen how important it is for those with Tinnitus to have their blood pressure checked regularly and to try to help themselves in this connection by undertaking seriously one of the relaxation disciplines. The reduction of stress in this way not only helps to lower blood pressure but is also without any side effects.

Chapter Sixteen

Insomnia

One of the worst of the various associated symptoms that follow Tinnitus is undoubtedly Insomnia.

My notes for this are headed 'Sleep ... The Drama of the Night' and drama it certainly is I can assure you, for there in the darkness of the night some very wonderful things happen to us all.

Our very earliest ancestors, the 'naked apes' who evolved from the original primates, would of course have been surrounded by enemies in a very hostile world. Nevertheless, at regular intervals they were obliged to go off guard and drift into sleep. This made them highly vulnerable within such dangerous surroundings, and so they chose the darkness in which to sleep, for it provided a cloak from their many enemies.

Sleep was just as vital to them as it is for us, their descendants; and so in spite of all the risks entailed it became an essential part of their biological rhythm which, evolving over millions of years has now become an essential element of our own lives.

Indeed, this sleep rhythm is now so fully established that it has been found that in cases where people have been imprisoned in caves and such-like, away from all social pressures, or changing light or darkness, and without watches or clocks, they will still fall into a pattern of sleep averaging eight hours or so in every twenty-four and closely allied to the light and dark of the outer world.

We are told that we can survive for over three weeks without food, but three weeks without sleep leaves one a mental and physical wreck. Thus sleep, like love, should never be taken for granted.

Habits of sleep are very much an individual matter. There are some people who can only function well on ten hours sleep a night, but most of us need much less than this.

With modern instruments much more has been learned lately

of the mysteries of sleep. For example, when we first close our eyes, our brain waves show a special rhythm of relaxation known as 'Alpha Rhythm'. As time goes on these waves become irregular as we begin to descend into a state of drowsiness known as 'Stage One Sleep'. At this stage the floating drift into sleep is often interrupted by what is known as the muscular 'Myoclonic Jerk' – a sudden muscular spasm of which one may or may not be aware.

In the past there have been a number of weird explanations and old wive's tales regarding the reason for the 'Myoclonic Jerk' I can recall at one lecture in my early teens being told that it was connected with the fact that since we all had evolved from a species which had possessed a prehensile tail (i.e. a tail capable of grasping) in the case of our ancestors who slept in trees this tail would sometimes slip and this sudden spasm or jerk still remained with us having been passed on in our genes. A likely theory perhaps, but even today the medical profession do not seem to be oversure of their own explanation which is that it is probably caused by the switching over of the brain from the conscious to the subconscious mind.

To continue . . . following the Myoclonic Jerk the muscles then relax, the heart slows down, and in about ten minutes we are into 'Stage Two Sleep'. In this stage our eyes roll slowly from side to side.

We later enter 'Stage Three Sleep' in which our muscles become relaxed, our breathing is even, and our heart rate, temperature and blood pressure all continue to drop fairly rapidly.

We then pass into the final stage of sleep known as 'Delta Sleep' or 'Stage Four Sleep'. At this point we are oblivious to any sounds which in the earlier stages could have awoken us.

We thus spend our nights in repeated descents and ascents throughout the four different stages of sleep. It is when we are in the ascending stage that the curtain rises on the most fascinating drama of the night . . . a drama in which you quite unknowingly take the leading role.

About an hour after we first fall asleep our eyes begin to make rapid jerky movements, these are uncannily co-ordinated as though we are watching something, and is quite unconnected with the unsynchronized rolling of the eyes during the initial period that I mentioned.

This particular phase of sleep is probably the best known, it is called 'Rapid Eye Movement' or 'REM' sleep'. In this the brain waves now resemble the waves found in the waking brain, and the heart rate and blood pressure become irregular, almost as if responding to some emotion or exertion.

With our oxygen consumption increasing at this stage it is as though our body is preparing for some immediate action. Curiously at this stage our muscles become slacker than in the other phases and our head and neck muscles lack support. Although seemingly geared for some immediate action, strangely enough it is at this very stage that it is most difficult to awaken anyone. The sleeper is now withdrawn. Withdrawn from the realities of life, and is actually living out a dream.

This direct association between REM Sleep and dreaming is one of the most important and exciting discoveries yet made in the field of sleep research, for it has opened up the way for a scientific study of dreaming.

And thus are all the old wive's tales about dreams swept away. For example it was seriously thought that dreams happened in a flash of time, but REM sleep-graphs show quite clearly that the time taken for playing out the action of a dream almost exactly matches the precise time that would be needed for the same action to occur during waking life.

Many people say that they never dream, and although they may well believe it, it is quite untrue. We all dream, but very quickly forget the essence of the dream. If we should by chance wake up and fully remember a vivid dream, then we have surfaced straight out of our REM sleep and this is why we are able to recall that dream.

The cycles of sleep I have described, leading up to the REM stage are repeated four or five times a night for all of us, within a normal eight hour period.

Curiously dreams can be influenced by external stimuli, proving that we are not completely cut off from the outside world whilst asleep. As an example drops of water sprinkled on a dreamer can lead them to dreaming of showers of rain. A humming noise can be interpreted by a dreamer as being a car in their dream. Actual bodily sensations or demands such as often do much toward helping a person to sleep, but above all a good bed is essential, and this is one feature that is so often overlooked. Surely since we spend something like one third of our lives in bed, the selection certainly deserves some thought.

The chief hazard and culprit of a poor night's sleep is all too often a sagging bed. This gives no support to the spinal muscles, and just rolls the sleeper into a most uncomfortable position in the middle. A bed that is too hard also hinders sleep for the simple reason that it does not cradle the body. Such a bed creates hollows at the waist and between the ribs and knees, making it impossible for those muscles to relax properly.

A correct bed is one which is pliable, and designed to follow the curves of the body whilst still giving ample support. The size of the bed is also important. A single bed should always be as wide as the distance between one's outstretched elbows and long enough to enable you to lie comfortably with your arms above your head. Not that this is a good position for the heart, but merely to check the bed length required.

For those with Tinnitus, the best method of overcoming Insomnia is to approach bedtime with a relaxed body and a quiet mind. A warm bath will help relax the body, and a short session of relaxation will help both body and mind. During the day try to get sufficient exercise and spend a while in the open air. Avoid a heavy meal or drinking very much for some three hours before retiring, and above all do not carry the worries of the day to bed with you.

At the expense of appearing unromantic I have to tell you that the experts inform us that anyone suffering from insomnia should sleep on their own; and have a room of their own. It is said that this gives an added freedom and generates a feeling of security both of which are vital to attaining perfect sleep. One paper I referred to on this matter had another angle; it said 'As to the question of is it best to sleep alone or with someone else. The answer is certainly sleep with someone else if their presence is a source of comfort to you . . . but if not SLEEP ALONE AT ALL COSTS!'

Chapter Seventeen

The Enigma of Tinnitus

Surely one of the main reasons for so little progress having been made in the study of Tinnitus lies in the fact that it is not possible to undertake research on something that cannot possibly be quantified, for it completely lacks any objective indicator.

It gives for example no fluctuation in temperature. No indications in the composition or chemistry of the blood, nor of the urine. Nor does it show anything whatever on X-ray film. All that the would-be researcher has before him is the actual report of the person claiming to experience Tinnitus. Unfortunately, to the scientific mind a report such as this which cannot be checked nor determined is completely unsatisfactory from the outset.

A further puzzling aspect of Tinnitus is in the fact that the reports of actual location of the noises can vary to such a great extent. Many who experience Tinnitus state that the sounds come from the ears, others that the noises seem to be at the back of the head. It can be in one ear or the other, or both, Some people have a different sound in one ear to the other. Occasionally one can come across people who are quite adamant that the noises are coming from an outside source and not from the head or ears at all. This has been described as 'pseudo tinnitus' yet the remarkable thing is that some of these people state they are hearing both tinnitus and this 'pseudo tinnitus' at the same time.

Those who cling to the idea of the noises originating from the environment can cause considerable problems to such authorities as Water Companies, Electricity Boards, Gas Companies and large factories etc. Others put the blame on Secret Military Testing, Space Experiments and so on. (See Chapter Eighteen)

The odd paradox of Tinnitus, be it from whatever source is surely the fact that although it is so very prevalent throughout the world, those suffering from it so rarely draw attention to it. It is only during the last decade or so that any publicity at all has been given to it, and yet still the medical profession can do little or nothing to alleviate it, let alone cure it.

One unfortunate and not infrequent consequence of a Tinnitus Patient presenting to a doctor with Tinnitus and at the same time showing obvious signs of depression – a symptom so often associated with it – is that certain anti-depressants may be prescribed. Unfortunately some of these actually list Tinnitus as a side effect with the result that the noises already depressing the patient are exacerbated further.

It is essential that anyone with Tinnitus presenting to their Doctor should acquaint him or any other practitioner that they may be referred to, that they suffer from Tinnitus. All too often people fail to do this. They are possibly nervous, or foolishly regard it as being socially unacceptable and therefore refrain from stating that they have Tinnitus.

There are numerous drugs that can influence neurotransmission without actual hearing loss and other drugs that may cause Tinnitus and Cochlear damage. A number of drugs can cause Tinnitus in anyone susceptible to it, and various ear, nose and eye drops, nasal sprays and ear ointments containing Neomycin which can have an ototoxic effect, as can aspirin or quinine.

It is a great pity that so many are so diffident in declaring that they suffer from Tinnitus, for more exposure of the problem would result in more public awareness of it, and this is something that is badly needed today.

TINNITUS AND THE TEETH

There is a relationship between the occlusion of the teeth and the temporomandibular (lower jaw) joint. When the occlusion of the teeth is wrong it can so easily lead to spasm in those muscles which control this joint. The muscles of the inner ear are also innervated by these same nerves and linked to these muscles via ligaments.

This explains why a poor occlusion of the teeth can so easily lead to spasms of the middle ear muscles and this can result in Tinnitus.

One method of overcoming the difficulty is by the fitting of an 'Occlusion Splint' made of hard thin plastic which disengages the teeth and tends to bring the lower jaw forward. Occasionally both an upper and lower splint may be fitted. Such splints can be easily removed by the wearer and are usually worn for a matter of from three to six months. If successful, then a permanent setting of the bite can be carried out.

Tests for this dysfunction should always be carried out with any tinnitus patient with whom it appears likely, but of course this particular dysfunction only applies to a very small proportion of those people experiencing Tinnitus.

Such dysfunction has been attributed to a number of causes apart from dental occlusion. It is said that it can be caused by chewing habits, stress or injury to a jaw joint. The latter can be caused by anything as simple as a yawn, sneeze or cough or by opening the mouth wide in order to bite a large object. It can also of course occur in any car or sporting accident.

Pain from the affected joint or joints involves local muscles and these can go into painful spasm as they try to avoid the joint moving. The effect of this can be one of pain in the face or jaws, headaches, eye aches, ear aches, pain in the neck and tongue and aching in the throat. It can even cause disturbances in one's vision and in the hearing and can often cause tinnitus.

Reports on treatment state that tinnitus arising from this problem can be eliminated or significantly reduced in some 50% of patients in which the joint/muscle disorder can be treated.

MEDICALLY RELATED CAUSES OF TINNITUS

We are all fairly aware of the usual causes of Tinnitus such as the degeneration of the hair cells of the cochlea, or the effects of the pathological mechanism of Meniere's Disease due to the increase in the amount of endolymph fluid in the inner ear. Most people are also aware of the effects of impacted wax against the ear drum, or of Otosclerosis which is caused by new bone formation affecting the little stapes or bones of the middle ear.

I would like to point out that in addition there are a number of causes which are medically related and not so often referred to.

As an example let us take Cervical Spondylosis which is the medical term for the degeneration changes in the upper segments of the backbone. With this, pressure is caused on the nerve roots that emerge between the vertebrae.

Similarly Arthritis inflaming as it does the tissues of joints, is also thought to play its part in the causation of Tinnitus. One difficulty here is that any drugs prescribed for arthritis are heavily slanted toward aspirin which can as we have seen in itself not only cause, but severely exacerbate an existing tinnitus.

Tinnitus can also occur as a symptom of several systemic diseases such as Multiple Sclerosis in which scattered areas of the brain and spinal cord degenerate and the nerve fibres lose their insulating sheath and thus their ability to conduct the electrical nerve pulses.

Paget's Disease is a gradual progressive bone disease characterized by bones breaking down through growing too rapidly and too thin, the bone being fragile and weak. In this blindness, hearing loss and Tinnitus can be caused by the skull pressing on the brain.

In America there is much made of Zinc Deficiency as likely to be a cause of tinnitus, but we hear little of this in the UK. So far as Tinnitus is concerned, zinc deficiency leads to anaemia, and anaemia is due to a shortage of the oxygen carrying pigment of the blood being in short supply. Pernicious anaemia is caused by a shortage of B12 vitamin, and tinnitus can often arise as a symptom.

The effects of thyroid disorder can also cause Tinnitus. Over-functioning leads to increased fuel consumption in the body, with irritability, restlessness and loss of weight. Under-functioning is characterised by loss of energy and appetite and dullness of the mind. Either can bring Tinnitus forward as a symptom.

In the later stages of Syphilis, Tinnitus can arise because it produces leaks between the various hitherto separate fluid systems in the inner ear.

By producing a reduction in middle ear compression Catarrh can also produce tinnitus. Even a very bad cold can cause a stiffness in the mechanism of the middle ear and set up Tinnitus.

Herpes Zoster, known more popularly as Shingles can also sometimes produce tinnitus as this virus is capable of producing deafness.

Migraine which is caused by too great a sensitivity in the blood vessels of the head is also thought to be a likely cause of Tinnitus, and one expert places this high on his priority list of things to be taken into account when first examining a patient presenting with Tinnitus.

A further factor likely to be a cause of Tinnitus is High Blood Pressure as this causes changes in the blood supply to the small vessels of the inner ear.

Since it is common knowledge that the structure of the ear and that of the kidney are closely linked, in any severe case of Tinnitus a test on Kidney Function should certainly be included.

Bell's Palsy, which is a complaint causing paralysis in the nerve at the side of the face, is said to be capable of producing Tinnitus. In this condition one of the two facial nerves swells up within its insulation and the wall of the canal constricts the swollen nerve. So often Tinnitus accompanies such a condition.

In concluding this short run-down of medical related factors I must of course add the very many drugs and antibiotics that actually list Tinnitus. Our hearing mechanism is one of the most sensitive parts of the body and Tinnitus can so often be tracked down to one of the many side effects of certain prescribed drugs.

METHODS OF AURAL HYGIENE

In normal circumstances ear wax (known as Cerumen) is being continually moved outwards by the action of the jaw bones and the natural shedding of our skin. This wax is made up of the oil secretions of the modified sweat glands in the outer part of the ear canal, plus scales from the skin and dust particles that have entered the canal.

It is quite harmless until with some people it starts to accumulate, when it can so easily cause temporary deafness. This accumulation is more likely to occur with people working in dusty occupations such as millers, carpenters or refuse collectors and so on. It can easily occur with those people having an excess of hair in the ears, or inflammation of the skin or scalp.

Any accumulation of wax may cause a variety of symptoms. Nine out of ten people then appear to do just the wrong things. They try to remove it with the aid of such things as matches, cotton wool buds, hairpins or any other such implements that may come to hand. The effect of this will most often be that the wax becomes impacted at the narrowest part of the ear canal which in itself can then cause irritation and often Tinnitus.

Sudden deafness can so often result from swimming or even

from taking a shower. This is caused by water entering the ear canal and swelling any wax that may be there. In such cases a person can additionally feel very dizzy.

The accepted method of wax removal has been syringing with warm water, the operator aiming the jet to the upper part of the ear canal so that it brings the wax forward and out. It is my firm opinion that such syringing should never be carried out on any person with tinnitus or susceptible to it. I know of many people who having presented to their Doctor with a wax problem and had their ears syringed in this way, have developed Tinnitus very soon afterwards. In fact it is a story that I hear repeatedly.

I fully appreciate that such syringing has been going on for many years and that in many cases it does not have this effect on a person, and am willing to accept that a pre-existing impairment in the auditory system can often be the underlying factor in the emergence of tinnitus, but the incidence of Tinnitus so quickly following syringing with so many people is to me extremely convincing; whilst at the same time freely admitting that many people have had this done quite frequently without any bad effect. For those of us with hearing impairment or existing Tinnitus it is surely better to be safe than sorry.

To avoid the possibility of this danger I would suggest you ask your GP to refer you to a Clinic or Specialist who has the necessary equipment and qualifications for your ears to be cleared by the "Suction Clearance Method". This is not something that your doctor can undertake.

I would certainly recommend that in all cases where wax has been neglected and accumulated in considerable quantity it is important that it should be dealt with by this method.

Those members who have had this treatment lately have reported on it most favourably as against the older method and some have even told me that it was quite pleasant. The patient lies on his or her back with the head on one side, the specialist looks into the ear with a microscope having high magnification and illumination. Then, using either a metal or plastic speculum (an instrument that holds the walls of the ear canal open) the ear is examined with the microscope. Any debris or wax can then be lifted out carefully with fine forceps and should soft wax exist this is drawn out by a small suction tube attached to a little vacuum pump.

Chapter Eighteen

The Phenomenon of Low Frequency Hums

What would cause an otherwise perfectly normal man to sleep on a local park bench during many of the late Spring and Summer nights? Or to camp out in the Market Square whilst his wife brings him food and drink during the day? The answer to this and much more lies in the Phenomenon of Low Frequency Noise, which is being reported by many thousands of people in this country. In this particular case this man's local park and his city centre are two locations he has discovered in which these mysterious noises do not trouble him.

This problem has been known for at least two decades yet still remains a mystery although the number of complaints have increased at an alarming rate.

It has been authoritatively stated that many thousands of people all over the country are complaining of being plagued by this noise. This may well be a very conservative estimate, for amongst a wealth of personal reports on my own files many of these people are stating that they find it best not to say anything to others about it in case they may be regarded as 'mad' or 'weird.' There must thus be a host of unreported cases.

Although not a sufferer, I personally became aware of the phenomenon around 1986 when the media reported a number of complaints of a low pitched humming sound in the small village of Worlingham in Suffolk. I am aware that there existed reports of this problem much earlier than this.

I spent a whole day in Worlingham at the time and interviewed a considerable number of these people. My tentative suggestion that perhaps some of them were suffering from a low frequency type of Tinnitus was met on all sides with adamant rejection. They were quite certain that the noise they were hearing was not in their head or ears but reaching them externally.

All were articulate, sensible people, and in no way 'cranky' or unusual. Of the people I interviewed there was a fairly even distribution of both men and women from all walks of life. Although I have had Tinnitus for many years, quite frankly I could hear nothing of the kind of noise they seemed to be experiencing, yet even as I spoke to them many were being obviously greatly disturbed by something.

It was at the time that my earlier book on Tinnitus was just going to the publishers and I felt that the problem was so closely allied to Tinnitus that I decided at almost the last minute to include a chapter on it in that book.

Possibly there have been no other published books dealing with this particular phenomenon since, but the outcome has been that I have received numerous reports on the matter not only from Britain but from several foreign countries as well.

I do not think that anyone would dispute the fact that this phenomenon exists and that everyone should be made aware of the fact that it is causing untold misery to many thousands of people. Yet despite many attempts no one has yet been able to trace the source and prove it. It has become popularly known as 'The Hum' and those suffering from it are known as 'Hummers'.

In 1989 these people, finding that nothing was being done except for spasmodic reports appearing in various newspapers etc from time to time and leading nowhere, formed their own Society in Britain known as The Low Frequency Noise Sufferers Association and today they appear to have a large membership. Not only do they keep in contact with each other by means of a regular newsletter, but I also know that many of them have their own private circles and these people regularly phone one another comparing intensities and other current features of the noise.

Numerous suggestions have been put forward at different times from various sources as to the cause, most popular being that the large underground pipe lines carrying North Sea Gas are to blame. The strength of this suggestion has often been apparently backed by the fact that increased incidence seems to occur soon after the laying of these pipe lines. But on this British

Gas reply 'It is one hundred per cent certain there is no link, We have done all sorts of tests on the whole theory'.

Other suggestions have revolved around such things as electricity pylons, water mains, underground railways and water pumps, generators, fans, transformers, electromagnetic fields set up around radio or TV transmitters, micro-waves, etc ... but nothing has been firmly identified as being the cause. Meantime thousands of sufferers are having the quality of their lives severely affected and feel extremely bitter that so little is being done to help them.

It is an interesting point that from a report of a Conference on 'The Hum' held at The Royal Society of Medicine, London, on the 25th of November 1989 it appears that the majority of people suffering from the problem state that the noise appears to have two differing components – a straight forward 'hum' plus another lower frequency modulation.

Sufferers report that the noise is quite unlike that of tinnitus as it does not emanate from within the head or ears and to many of them it appears to reach them through walls, floors and ceilings when inside the house, and externally when outside. It causes them considerable stress and loss of sleep which greatly lowers the quality of their life. The long-term effects of such exposure have yet to be documented.

One sufferer who lives in Romsey says 'I don't know what I am living for. I can get no rest and I stalk the house at night weeping with the effects. I feel like a caged animal, exhausted and hopeless, dejected and demotivated'. She has been a successful professional Artist and has been obliged to give up her work completely as she 'crumbles against the relentless effects of this torturing Hum.'

A sufferer from Leicester whose two daughters and herself are all suffering badly from the noise writes 'at all hours of the day and night we roam around the area trying to locate the source'. Being unable to sleep in the house when the noise is particularly bad, she is forced to sleep in the garden shed, the only place in her home where she is free of the problem. This sufferer after approaching all the usual sources in vain wrote to the Ombudsman and received the following reply: 'The noise which causes you such personal disturbance is not sufficiently loud to constitute a statutory nuisance.' The fact that she reports the noise to be as loud as a normal television set appears to have been overlooked.

Although many of the usual Authorities concerned in such matters certainly do seem to try to research the matter within their own particular sphere, one can understand their not being particularly pleased by any such accusations, for the realisation must always be with them that should they be found to be the culprit, correction could well be a very expensive business.

This phenomenon is not by any means confined to Britain for I personally know that it exists in Italy, Canada and Spain and probably worldwide.

It is imperative that everyone should keep an open mind on this matter and not jump to conclusions without considerable weighing up of the pros and cons.

There are a number of very good reasons why these people should be taken seriously. It is all too easy to point to the possibilities of some aural dysfunction – this is the standard explanation from most of the medical profession. But it is pointed out that these sufferers from 'the Hum' are able to find certain places in which they do not experience the noise at any time. This is very different from the experience of anyone with tinnitus in which the noises are with them wherever they may be.

Additionally a number of these people will tell you that they also have tinnitus and are quite aware that one noise is within the head and the other definitely coming from some external source.

It seems to me that one very reasonable explanation might be that certain people may have an extension of the normal spectrum of hearing, and if this extension leans toward the lower range of frequencies they may well be picking up some noise which others cannot hear as it is beyond the range of normal hearing.

There have been reports of 'Hummers' going into deep limestone caves such as exist in Cheddar and Wookey Hole when the noise completely ceases – a further indication that this is no fantasy.

Whilst Noise Experts admit to being completely baffled, thousands of people continue to suffer from the phenomenon and are being made ill by untraceable sounds which the other members of their families cannot hear at all.

Their only hope is that pressure of public opinion will in time stimulate more research into this phenomenon and so help to release them from a life which is little more than a living Hell at present.

I feel that what is needed most of all at the moment is for the three professional camps involved – the Authorities, the Medical World and the Noise Experts to agree to pool knowledge and resources in a combined effort to try to pin down the cause whether it be medical or factual and thus help thousands of people many of whom are at the end of their tether.

Looking Ahead

What of the future? It has only been during the last decade or so that any really concentrated efforts have been made in the research and study of Tinnitus, and it is encouraging now to see such work going on in most countries of the world to some degree or other.

Most people with Tinnitus are puzzled and impatient by so little real progress being made in this connection but this mainly lies in the fact that it is so extremely difficult to study something that cannot be quantified nor measured, and completely lacks any objective indicator.

A popular remark in Tinnitus circles in the USA. is "For Tinnitus there seems to be no magic bullet but Oh Boy! there's plenty of Buckshot!"

And how true this is. Looking back over the fairly recent past alone we have witnessed a number of seemingly exciting prospects of cure, all of which have proved useless under strict testing. In many of these cases no sooner do we read of some extremely exciting experiment, falsely raising everyones hopes yet again, than we hear it has gone to the wall like all the rest.

As to the possibilities of cure, my personal feeling is that very probably as Research continues (and even as I write there are several very sensible such channels being explored) perhaps some new discovery will help to at least alleviate – or possibly cure – just one of the many types of Tinnitus; and as time goes on possibly relief or cure will be found for other causes.

Let this be our constant hope.

LESLIE SHEPPARD